Leadership and Communication in Dentistry

Leadership and Communication in Dentistry

A Practical Guide to Your Practice,
Your Patients, and Your Self

Joseph P. Graskemper

Clinical Associate Professor,
Stony Brook School of Dental Medicine,
Stony Brook,
NY, USA

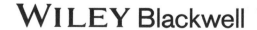

This edition first published 2019

© 2019 John Wiley and Sons, Inc

The right of Joseph P. Graskemper to be identified as the author of this work has been asserted in accordance with law.

Registered Office
John Wiley & Sons, Inc., 111 River Street, Hoboken, NJ 07030, USA

Editorial Office
111 River Street, Hoboken, NJ 07030, USA

For details of our global editorial offices, customer services, and more information about Wiley products visit us at www.wiley.com.

Wiley also publishes its books in a variety of electronic formats and by print-on-demand. Some content that appears in standard print versions of this book may not be available in other formats.

Library of Congress Cataloging-in-Publication Data

Names: Graskemper, Joseph P., author.
Title: Leadership and communication in dentistry: a practical guide to your practice,
    your patients and your self / Joseph P. Graskemper.
Description: Hoboken, NJ: Wiley-Blackwell, 2019. | Includes bibliographical
    references and index. |
Identifiers: LCCN 2018054061 (print) | LCCN 2018055297 (ebook) | ISBN 9781119557142
    (AdobePDF) | ISBN 9781119557135 (ePub) | ISBN 9781119557210 (paperback)
Subjects: | MESH: Interpersonal Relations | Practice Management, Dental |
    Leadership | Communication | Insurance, Dental | Dentists–psychology
Classification: LCC RK58.5 (ebook) | LCC RK58.5 (print) | NLM WU 61 |
    DDC 617.60068–dc23
LC record available at https://lccn.loc.gov/2018054061

Cover Design: Wiley
Cover Images:© Beautiful landscape/Shutterstock, © Martin Barraud/Getty Images

Set in 10/12pt Warnock by SPi Global, Pondicherry, India

Printed in the United States of America

V10008517_022819

Contents

Preface

This book is the result of many recent dental school graduates seeking advice regarding the direction their careers and their lives were heading. Some lost the balance required to maintain a healthy practice and a healthy home life. Some would mention after our sessions on leadership that they never heard of such material and wished they had more information. To maintain your life is not only to be living successfully but also to be successful at living. In dentistry, we need to take the lead in our involvement in dental insurance, or in our practices as it relates to our patients and our staffs, and the lead on how we manage ourselves to maintain that leadership and maintain our life. Communication goes hand in hand with leadership, and therefore this book gives great attention to how we communicate with those we lead. It is understandable that many dental schools do not have enough scheduled time in the education of future dentists to allot significant time to communication and leadership. This book presents the basic understanding of communication and leadership in the dental practice.

There are many instances when written communication is a must. A written communication is often a memorialization of what was said or to convey or make known one's thoughts, reasonings, and beliefs. All great leaders have based their leadership on great communication. There are basically four stakeholders in dentistry: insurance companies (payers), patients, staff, and dentists (providers). Dentists must constantly communicate with insurance companies, patients, and staff. Dentists must also lead the insurance discussion to maintain a successful practice, lead patients to become motivated, lead staff to perform properly, and lead the direction of their life to be self-dedicated and keep focused on their self and their families. Each requires an individualized communication regarding a variety of issues. What must be said to a dental insurance company in advocacy for your patient is very different than what is communicated to your staff/ employees and again different to one's self to maintain leadership. Being mindful of proper communication and leadership skills create a true balance for the successful dentist leader. Therefore, this book has been divided into three sections: Dental Insurance Companies, Your Practice, which includes patients and staff, and Your Self.

My first book, *Professional Responsibility In Dentistry: A Practical Guide to Law and Ethics*, had to deal with the legal, ethical, and practice management issues that dentists face in their professional careers. Like my first book there are True Case/Examples in this book to help illustrate a point or concept. It should be pointed out that many of the suggestions, concepts, and illustrations may need to be adapted to your jurisdiction's rules, regulations, and laws; and you should always retain proper legal, tax, and practice management advice when applicable.

Acknowledgments

I dedicate this book to my wife, Tara, who is always there and supportive of my pursuits. She is my confidant, my sounding board, and the only person who keeps me balanced in my life. She is my companion who is at my side whenever needed. My love is beyond that which can be said with words. And "Yes," I will get all the "book stuff" off the kitchen table.

I also want to acknowledge my children and their spouses for their encouragement and support while they are all balancing their lives and following their roads to be successful at living. Thank you to Joey and his wife Allie, Gena and her husband Eric, and Paige. You are all special to me. I appreciate your patience and understanding while I took on this endeavor, often times caught up in thought.

And to my office staff, Michele Yalamas RDH, Erin Condit RDH, Cathy Perten, Susan Sawyer, and Sandra Richiusa for all your understanding and constantly hearing: "Just a minute, I need to finish this thought" or "I'll be right there," only to be reminded 10 minutes later.

I would also like to acknowledge those whom I may not have identified sooner and from whom I have drawn my conclusions and opinions and apologize in advance of any inadvertent omission.

Author's Note

This work is sold with the understanding that the author is not engaged in rendering professional services such as, but not limited to, legal or tax advice. The advice or strategies contained herein may not be suitable to your situation and therefore you should always seek professional advice in your jurisdiction.

Acknowledgments

I dedicate this book to my wife, Tara, who is always there and supportive of my pursuits. She is my confidant, my sounding board, and the only person who keeps me balanced in my life. She is my companion who is at my side whenever needed. My love is beyond that which can be said with words. And "Yes," I will get all the "book stuff" off the kitchen table.

I also want to acknowledge my children and their spouses for their encouragement and support while they are all balancing their lives and following their roads to be successful at living. Thank you to Joey and his wife Allie, Gena and her husband Eric and Paige. You are all special to me. I appreciate your patience and understanding while I took on this endeavor, often times caught up in thought.

And to my office staff, Michele Yalamas RDH, Erin Condit RDH, Cathy Perten, Susan Sawyer, and Sandra Richluso for all your understanding and constantly insisting (Just a minute, I need to finish this thought" or "I'll be right there," only to be reminded 10 minutes later.

I would also like to acknowledge those whom I may not have identified sooner and from whom I have drawn my conclusions and opinions and apologize in advance of any inadvertent omission.

Section 1

Leadership and Success in Communication with Dental Insurance Companies

With the continuing intrusion into the practice of dentistry, dentists must have a full understanding of the insurance company's provider agreements, dental care limitations, and policy manuals; thereby, allowing the dentist to become an advocate for the patient and be successful in his or her dental practice.

Leadership and Communication in Dentistry, First Edition. Joseph P. Graskemper.
© 2019 John Wiley & Sons, Inc. Published 2019 by John Wiley & Sons, Inc.

1

Understanding Insurance Companies

Let no feeling of discouragement prey upon you,
and in the end you are sure to succeed.
Abraham Lincoln

Our doubts are traitors, and make us lose we oft might win,
by fearing to lose.
Shakespeare

Whether you accept dental insurance or not, you as a dental office owner must master certain communication skills to properly provide care for those patients with insurance coverage. Dental insurance has made such an impact on the patient's perspective of how they choose their dental care that it directly or indirectly affects all dental offices. Therefore, this section presents basic understanding and some sample letters for proper communication on a wide variety of dental insurance issues. Dental insurance companies have become a major stakeholder in dental healthcare. Beginning in the 1950s and really blossoming in the 1970s, insurance companies are now a major payer for dental services. Dental insurance, like all other insurances, was intended to be a help for patients to obtain needed dental work. Dentists even founded their own dental insurance company called Delta Dental. Dental insurance was never meant to be the full payer or overseer of dental care. However, corporate profits do change viewpoints resulting in corporate control of how, when, and where dental care is provided. With this intrusion into the doctor–patient relationship and having a focus on making a profit for their shareholders, insurance companies have exerted more and more control over the procedures that would be covered, and if, how, and when those procedures will be paid for. Even though the insurance company makes the rules, we can take the lead in making the rules work for us, our practices, and our patients. We must take control of this intrusion through proper advocacy for our patients.

Leadership and Communication in Dentistry, First Edition. Joseph P. Graskemper.
© 2019 John Wiley & Sons, Inc. Published 2019 by John Wiley & Sons, Inc.

First you have to understand the insurance conundrum to better communicate with insurance companies just like understanding your patient's needs and wants to better communicate with them.

It is a conundrum because the insurance companies exist primarily to make a profit for its shareholders while providing health services to trusting clients, who expect untethered coverage. The term "insurance companies" includes self-administered and self-funded dental coverage. Some jurisdictions do not apply insurance company rules and regulations to self-administered or self-funded dental coverage plans. As always seek proper legal advice regarding your state's policies, rules, and regulations. To make the system work, there are procedure limits and yearly monetary limits regardless of patient needs. However, we must work together for our patients and our mutual survival. Merely saying you do not work with dental insurance companies is not being realistic for most dentists.

Briefly, there are basically two types (exclusive of government-supported programs such as Medicaid) of insurance managed care, Health Maintenance Organization (HMO) and Preferred Provider Organization (PPO), with there being several types of both. The major difference between all plans is the manner in which the dentist is paid. There are also many other stipulations in the contract that are beyond the fee structure. An HMO often referred to as a capitation plan when it pays the dentist a monthly fee for each client/patient assigned to the dentist whether or not the patient comes to the office for dental care. In turn, the dentist will provide needed dental care with no further cost to the insurance company and at little to no cost to the patient. The less treatment provided or even if the patient does not come for appointments, the dentist makes a larger profit. This clearly puts pressure on the dentist to provide the least costly alternative treatment (LCAT) rather than the ideal treatment the patient may need or want. It also may create an ethical practice management dilemma of the duty to provide insurance-covered treatment and the loss of income.

There are several PPO formats. One, which I call Full PPO, has a PPO fee structure based on an agreed-upon reduced fee schedule that is paid in full by the insurance company. There is also the Percentage PPO, which has a fee structure based on an agreed-upon reduced fee schedule that is paid in part by the insurance company and in part by the patient, each paying their percentage of the full agreed-upon fee depending on the treatment provided. The Patient PPO is based on an agreed-upon reduced fee schedule that is paid in full by the patient.

Per the ADA survey, 73% of dental patients have some type of dental insurance, and 92.7% of dentists have contracted with two or more PPOs [1]. This clearly indicates the depth of dental insurance into the individual dentist's office.

Having provided dental care for patients for over 40 years, the impact of dental insurance companies has grown such that most dentists have experienced the impact of the dental consultant on the doctor–patient relationship and the decision-making process to provide their patients with optimal dental care.

Prior to dental insurance, there was only the doctor and the patient, relying on the doctor–patient relationship to determine the treatment to be rendered and how it would be paid for. It would be a mutually agreed-upon treatment from which the patient would receive optimum dental care without any intrusion from outside their doctor–patient relationship. It would give the patient autonomy in their decisions regarding their dental care. Now, insurance companies, being the major payer for dental care, want to have a say in what treatment will be rendered and how it will be paid for. Not being physically in the operatory to partake in the doctor–patient discussion and treatment decisions, they must rely on an ever-increasing need of information to substantiate and verify that treatment was needed and completed. The final decision making on how a patient should be cared for is and should continue to be between the doctor and the patient. Hence, the dentist must fully understand insurance companies and how to work with this unavoidable intrusion into the doctor–patient relationship to provide proper care for their patients.

Contrary to the common belief that dental insurance has lowered the cost of dental care, it has actually increased it. By issuing a lower contracted fee schedule and requiring more dental office staff time to verify the patient's eligibility, submit a predetermination, resubmit with additional documentation, reverify eligibility, resubmit for payment, and process bulk checks for numerous patients, insurance coverage has increased the cost of providing dental care. Compare this to a patient merely paying in full at the end of each visit. To help cover the additional costs of accepting dental insurance, which many times includes hiring another employee, the dentist's Usual, Customary, and Reasonable (UCR) fee must be increased to offset losses incurred by accepting dental insurance or risk reducing income and/or insolvency. Hence, the non-insured patients must pay higher UCR fees to offset the lower insured fees.

The dentist, if accepting insurance as a panel or listed dentist, must understand his or her duties to the patient do not change. The dentist, adhering to the ADA Code of Ethics, should be aware of patient autonomy, non-malfeasance, beneficence, justice, and veracity. The proposed treatment must not cause harm to the patient and must improve the patient's well-being. Many times, the insurance company will provide coverage for the LCAT per the policy. Being an insurance-accepting dentist creates a relationship whereby the dentist must be open to treatment alternatives and not offer only the most optimum treatment that is outside of insurance coverage. Maintaining the patient's autonomy throughout the decision-making process is paramount in maintaining a healthy, trusting doctor–patient relationship. The standard of care must also be considered when allowing the insurance company's LCAT policy to rule over patient care. If the proposed LCAT is not in the patient's best interests and/or below the standard of care, the dentist should appeal it or simply not provide the substandard care, even if the patient wants it due to lowered costs. To do so would expose the treating dentist to a possible lawsuit for malpractice by providing substandard care. The dentist may not point to the insurance company for liability due to the fact the dentist actually provided the treatment. Hence, if the LCAT is not within the standard of care, the dentist must refuse to provide such treatment even if the patient agrees to it.

The dentist also needs to have a better understanding of business decisions needed to become involved in dental insurance due to the fact that some dental insurance fee schedules are very unreasonable and not conducive to proper patient care. These should obviously be discarded so as not to force a dentist into a standard of care issue. When the unilateral "take it or leave it contract" is presented to the dentist, it contains a "negotiated" fee schedule. The dentist normally reviews the fee schedule, besides other aspects of the contract (of which nothing can be changed or rarely negotiated), and decides whether to accept it or not. (The ADA has a contract review service available. As with any contract, seek proper local legal advice prior to signing the provider agreement.) However, when the pre-authorization or claim is submitted and it is denied due to being a non-covered service, even though it is on their agreed-upon fee schedule, the dentist must still abide by the fee schedule even though the insurance company does not. This occurs because of their pursuit of increased profits by not paying their fair share. Some states have or are in the process of making such practices unlawful. These types of laws are often referred to as "anti-fee capping laws" or "fee capping laws." They vary widely as to their scope of regulation. Some insurance provider contracts state that certain dental procedures may not be referred to a specialist and paid only if the general dentist, though not proficient, performs the treatment to accommodate the patient [2]. In other words, the dentist is forced to do procedures he or she is not trained or not proficient to do, resulting in an ethical, financial, and possibly legal dilemma for the dentist. The dentist should turn to the ADA Code of Ethics regarding patient autonomy, non-malfeasance, and beneficence and review risk management protocols before proceeding with treatment contractually dictated by the insurance company that may be beyond his or her scope or limitations of practice.

It should be pointed out that the dentist is under no obligation to sign a dental insurance company's contract and work under it, nor is the dentist and patient obliged to provide treatment only within the dental insurance company's coverage levels. The dentist and the patient always have the option to not work within the dental insurance framework. Nevertheless, dental insurance is here and will continue to grow in the dental healthcare system, affecting many decisions regarding patient care.

Rather than just two shareholders, the doctor and the patient, to decide treatment, now there are four shareholders having interests in the patient's dental care: 1) the patient, 2) the dentist, 3) the consultant, and 4) the insurance company. Each not only has a financial interest but should also have an ethical interest to seek the best care for the patient.

Not all dentists need to be involved with insurance and should make a personal decision whether to be involved in the patient's insurance coverage or not. The dentist is under no duty to accept insurance involvement in his or her practice, but the patient must be made aware of that office policy decision prior to providing treatment. A fully informed patient includes the costs of the procedure with or without insurance coverage per the patient's situation. For more on informed consent, see *Professional Responsibility in Dentistry: A Practical Guide to Law and Ethics*, chapter 8.

The dentist has the duty to provide treatment within the standard of care. To submit claims for substandard care is a breach of that duty to the patient regardless of any type of insurance coverage the patient may have. Hence, the dentist has a duty to submit only for treatment that is within the standard of care and fulfilling basic treatment protocols. To maintain the patient's autonomy, the dentist also has a duty to provide the patient with the information necessary to make an informed decision, including cost, regarding the treatment proposed regardless of whether it is or is not a covered procedure.

The costs should be broken down as to the insurance portion and the patient portion so the patient is fully informed regarding their financial responsibilities. Therefore, if the dentist becomes involved in dental insurance, he/she or staff should have a firm understanding of the policy coverage limitations to properly discuss treatment options within and outside of coverage for a valid informed consent. Due to patients not understanding treatment codes and dental terminology, the dentist also takes on the additional ethical obligation to be the patient's advocate to obtain the best treatment possible under the insurance guidelines with proper documentation, if the patient so desires. The doctor–patient relationship, being fiduciary, demands the dentist to keep the patient's autonomy (the right to self-determination) and the concepts of malfeasance (do no harm) and beneficence (patient well-being) ethically intact. This can be easily done by submitting a predetermination for benefits and receiving an Estimation of Benefits (EOB). Once the treatment plan has been finalized via a full discussion and a proper informed consent, the proposed treatment plan should be sent to the insurance company with complete documentation that should include periodontal charting, necessary radiographs, correct treatment codes, and a short written reason for any major treatment such as periodontal surgery, crown and bridge, and removable prosthodontics. A short narrative, one line long, on the claim form is usually sufficient to deflect any rejections and complete the documentation needed to expedite the claim review process. Upon receiving the EOB, the dentist may then properly inform the patient of the cost of treatment, which is a very large determining factor for most patient's decision-making process. By knowing the cost of treatment, the patient may properly exercise their autonomy and make an informed decision. Remember the EOB is only an estimate and is not a guarantee for payment. There are cases in which the insurance company has decided unilaterally not to honor their own EOB. There are many ways to provide financing for the patient, which is beyond the scope of this section (see Chapter 8).

True Case (1)

A patient presented with a fractured posterior tooth and needed a full coverage crown. The patient was very concerned about the cost because she had limited financial ability to pay the entire fee without her insurance. The dentist, having contracted with that particular insurance company, agreed to send in a predetermination for the benefit of the patient to find out the amount that the patient would have to pay. Upon receiving the Estimation of Benefits (EOB) form, the patient was informed of her patient portion and an appointment was made. When the procedure was then billed, the insurance company did not pay stating that their consultant now decided that an amalgam restoration was all that was needed and therefore the benefit paid was only for a three-surface amalgam. It also stated that the EOB is only an estimation and not a commitment. The dentist wrote an appeal letter and eventually received the proper dental benefits. (A sample letter can be found in Chapter 5.)

If the insurance company denies coverage or alters the treatment plan per the insurance policy guidelines to an alternative treatment, the patient should still be properly informed of all treatment options to maintain his or her autonomy. A full discussion on informed consent may be found in chapter 8, *Professional Responsibility in Dentistry: A Practical Guide to Law and Ethics* [3]. A denial of insurance coverage should be based on one of the following reasons: 1) not a covered service under the policy or exceeds the yearly maximum benefit, 2) improper or missing documentation, and 3) a less costly alternative treatment available per the policy. It is very understandable that all dental services may not be covered by the insurance policy. This does not mean that the patient is not entitled to the treatment beyond insurance coverage that his or her dentist has recommended or provided. Some denials may be hard to overcome since the dental consultant must adjudicate the claim per the patient's policy limitations. It should not be based on an individual consultant's treatment biases, if the consultant is following the American Association of Dental Consultants (AADC) Code of Ethics. Maintaining the patient's autonomy throughout the decision-making process is paramount in maintaining a healthy, trusting doctor–patient relationship.

Recently there have been some changes in the manner insurance companies have dealt with their dental providers. They have in the past only denied benefits for the patient. Now they have placed clauses in the contract stating that they can disallow treatment for their patient/client. This means that the dental provider, if they have signed such a contract, would not be allowed to provide the recommended treatment and if they did provide such treatment could not seek payment from the patient. I do not see how this new twist from the insurance companies could possibly continue.

Many dentists blame the insurance company's dental consultant for not allowing treatment for the patient when, in fact, the dental consultant, when following the AADC Code of Ethics, merely reviews treatment as to whether it is a viable treatment plan within the insurance company's benefits guidelines. If the LCAT plan is considered below the standard of care by the treating dentist, he or she is best to refuse providing such treatment and discuss with the patient a viable option. Although there is increased time and effort to become an advocate for your patient, the rewards of patient appreciation and the collateral referrals of non-covered patients (family and friends) are of benefit to the dentist.

The dental consultant is hired by the insurance company to review treatment plans submitted by the dentist to the insurance company for benefits under the policy the patient/client purchased. They are not all the same. There are many levels of dental coverage that may be purchased by the patient or his/her employer. The dental consultant determines whether treatment falls within the policy limitations. Most dental consultants are practicing dentists or have practiced dentistry for a minimum of five years per the AADC. As with all professions, all cannot be the best and all are not the worst. Sometimes faced with incomplete records submitted to provide treatment or secure a payment, the consultant must attempt to decide whether such incomplete records support the treatment and fall within the individual's policy guidelines. As a general rule, the consultant cannot make assumptions, but must adjudicate the claim based solely on the documents provided and within the dental benefit plan/policy guidelines.

The dental consultant has duties to the patient and the dental insurance company. The consultant, according to the AADC, has a duty and is "obliged to report to the appropriate reviewing agency evidence of impairment, illegal or unethical behavior on the part of the provider or peer" [4]. They also "should abide by the American Dental Association Code of Ethics" [3]. The duties owed to the patient according to the AADC Code of Ethics may be found in Principle 3: Beneficence:

> The dental consultant has a duty to promote the welfare of the patient, provider, peer and employer to the best of his or her ability within the limits of his contractual obligations.
>
> 3E. All dental consultants should abide by the American Dental Association Code of Ethics.
>
> 4A. The decisions a dental consultant makes are subject to the same ethical, moral, and educational standards used in the direct treatment of patients.

4B. The ethical aspects of dental consultant duties must always take precedence over economic aspects.

4C. The doctor patient relationship, even indirect, is fiduciary and must take precedence over economic or personal influences.

4D. The dental consultant must regard 'standard of care' the same for all providers.

(And lastly,) 10A. The dental consultant should strive to assist patients, providers, peers and employers in receiving and delivering the highest quality care available under the terms and guidelines of a particular contract. [2]

The AADC Code of Ethics further states: "The dental consultant should make every effort not to interfere with the doctor-patient relationship unless such relationship could jeopardize the public health or cause harm to a specific patient" [3]. Without the proper documentation to support the proposed treatment, the dental consultant has no other choice but to request more information, provide coverage for the LCAT, or refuse benefits. A refusal of benefits is not and should not be implied by the dentist that the submitted treatment plan is wrong, below the standard of care, or not in the patient's best interest. The least costly treatment alternative or refusal of coverage is merely a consultant's opinion that the proposed treatment is not within the dental insurance company's contractual benefit limitations or policy guidelines.

Therefore, the dental consultant, with proper documentation, has a duty to the patient to allow a level of treatment within the standard of care under the agreed-upon dental insurance contract and should allow benefit coverage.

The consultant also has duties to the dental insurance company. The AADC Code of Ethics points out:

3A. The dental consultant should work toward the goals of the company or the entity that employs said consultant and enforce the parameters of the policies issued by the body including its specific code of ethics.

3B. The dental consultant reviews strangers; (also known as unknown patients). It is said consultant's ethical duty to these strangers to view that brief and indirect relationship as one in which he or she is encouraged to do the most good for them as possible within the context of the plan and the standards of care relating to the proposed treatment.

Principle 6: Fidelity ('Honor your commitments') The dental consultant shall abide by the rules of his or her employer. [3]

Having a duty to fulfill their employer's rules and enforce the given parameters of the policy, the consultant may at times be restrained from allowing benefits for a desired treatment plan. The consultant in following company policies must allow only benefits for the LCAT. For example, the number of missing teeth in an arch may determine whether to allow for fixed or removable prosthodontics. Hence, it is not the consultant but the framework within which he or she must function that causes friction to develop between dentist and consultant. Therefore, it is of utmost importance to submit all supporting documentation, including any narratives necessary, as previously discussed, for the consultant to allow proper benefits based on your patient advocacy.

The consultant also has the problem of continued submission of substandard documentation and/or obvious questionable treatment plans from the same provider. There are also the submissions of fraudulent claims that may range from incidental (simple clerical mistakes) to serious (multiple root canal therapy on nonexistent teeth or submission for treatment not actually performed). The occasional incorrect billing or clerical mistake is usually and easily rectified by requesting more information or documentation to support the pre-authorization or claim. The ethical submitting doctor would be more likely than not be happy to correct the mistake and/or resubmit the requested documentation. It is the continued submission of seriously questionable claims from the same doctor that places the consultant between the proverbial "rock and a hard place." When such situations arise where the consultant must fulfill his or her duty to the insurance company and the patient, he or she must question multiple substandard claims from the same provider. Such an accusation should be supported by three elements as pointed out in the AADC Code of Ethics and the ADA Code of Ethics. The AADC lists the three elements as follows:

1) Dissent – The dental consultant must weigh the potential harm to future patients treated by the provider in question or harm caused by case review by the consultant in question. The following questions must then be answered: How accurate is the information? What will produce the most good with the least harm? Have all existing and less drastic avenues for change been tried in a timely manner?
2) Disloyalty – The dental consultant must ask the question: "Am I being excessively loyal to the patient, the provider, my fellow consultant, or my employer?"
3) Accusation – The dental consultant must ask the questions: "What are my motives? Do I have a vested interest in this case? Is the criticism justified and supported by scientific literature? Does a pattern exist or is this an isolated case?" [3]

The ADA Code of Ethics (which the dental consultant must also adhere to per 3E of the AADC Code) points out:

> 4.C. Justifiable Criticism. Dentists shall be obliged to report to the appropriate reviewing agency as determined by the local component or constituent society instances of gross or continual faulty treatment by other dentists. Patients should be informed of their present oral health status without disparaging comment about prior services. Dentists issuing a public statement with respect to the profession shall have a reasonable basis to believe that the comments made are true.
>
> C.1. Meaning of "Justifiable." Patients are dependent on dentists to know their oral health status. Therefore, when informing a patient of the status of his or her oral health, the dentist should exercise care that the comments made are truthful, informed and justifiable. This may involve consultation with the previous treating dentist, to determine under what circumstances and conditions the treatment was performed. A difference of opinion as to preferred treatment should not be communicated to the patient in a manner which would unjustly imply mistreatment. There will necessarily be cases where it will be difficult to determine whether the comments made are justifiable. Therefore, this section is phrased to address the discretion of dentists and advises against unknowing or unjustifiable disparaging statements against another dentist. However, it should be noted that, where comments are made which are not supportable and therefore unjustified, such comments can be the basis for the institution of a disciplinary proceeding against the dentist making such statements. [5]

Depending on the manner and the extent a dentist comments on a prior treating dentist, such statements may open the avenue to a lawsuit alleging defamation.

The dental consultant is therefore held to the duty to report continued substandard claims to the proper agency to primarily protect the patient and to fulfill his or her contractual obligations. This duty relates to claims and not proposed treatment plans submitted for predetermination/pre-estimate of benefits. Questionable treatment plans should simply be denied because the dental consultant cannot suggest or dictate treatment. It is beyond the scope of their employment to review submitted treatment plans as to being proper treatment or not. Rather it is whether the claim is within policy guidelines. It is a personal ethical choice of the dental consultant to report or personally call the dentist in question to allow the dentist to explain any extenuating circumstances that may have affected the treatment plan or claim in question. It is possible that some consultants who have brought attention to continued substandard claims to the insurance company have found that the company is hesitant to report further to the appropriate agency for fear of lawsuits. Some insurance companies have simply, but hesitantly, removed the dentist from their panel of insurance-accepting dentists. This is usually done without reason by merely relying on the contract to not renew it or give contractual notice (usually 60 or 90 days) that the contract will not be renewed. Reasons, again, are rarely given for fear of a costly lawsuit. In some states, insurance companies vigorously report continued questionable practices, especially if the situation involves upcoding or other fraudulent acts.

The dental insurance company has a duty primarily to the patient but also to its shareholders. Both place pressure on the insurance company to provide benefits (expenses) and to keep benefit claims within actuarial forecasts (profits). As a result of paying premiums, the patient trusts that the insurance company will provide benefits for the proposed treatment that was agreed to with the dentist. The acceptance of insurance premiums creates a duty on the insurance company to not withhold benefits for properly documented proposed treatment or claims for treatment that fall within the policy guidelines. To set guidelines for payment of benefits that make it next to impossible for the patient to receive those benefits is unconscionable. All stakeholders are aware that there are many levels of dental insurance coverage whereby some patients may have insurance that allows benefits for all dental treatment while others have very limiting policies. However, the insurance company must not withhold benefits that are properly submitted within the policy guidelines for the sole purpose of profits. Many states have laws that do not allow insurance companies to unreasonably delay adjudication of a claim. To not process a preauthorization in a timely manner is unethical, possibly causing harm to the patient by the delay, and possibly illegal, depending on the various states' laws.

If a dental office has a history of continued questionable or fraudulent claims, the insurance companies generally want suspect offices to be "red flagged" and ultimately routed to the legal department. Most times the dentist will be warned to cease and desist their questionable actions or be removed from the insurance company's list of providers as was previously mentioned.

True Case (2)

Many years ago, it was taught to place calcium hydroxide to all exposed dentin to protect the dentin from acid etching. The dentist would bill for the placement of the calcium hydroxide to cover the cost of the materials. The insurance company eventually sent a certified letter to the dentist to cease and desist from placing the indirect pulp cap under bonded composite restorations. The dentist then stopped such practice. Two years later the dentist was sued by a patient for practicing below the standard of care for not placing the calcium hydroxide under the composite restoration and resulted in a root canal per the plaintiff's expert witness. The case was settled in favor of the dentist.

Several other questionable practices that dental insurance companies have utilized for the sake of profits are the following: 1) bundling of procedures, 2) not raising yearly limits, 3) not covering procedures listed on their fee schedules, and 4) interfering in the doctor–patient relationship.

Being a practicing dentist for over 40 years, I, like others, have experienced the continued reduction of benefits by some insurance companies utilizing questionable unilateral bundling decisions. Some insurance companies bundle procedures together to reduce the reimbursement to the dentist and the benefit to the patient to increase their profits, which allow shareholders to enjoy a better return on investment. Commonly bundled procedures are the placement of pins being added and made part of the buildup procedure and then making buildups part of the crown procedure, making fluoride treatments part of a prophylaxis, and making pulp-cap procedure part of the restoration. This creates an ethical dilemma for the dentist whether to provide free treatment under the insurance guidelines.

The yearly maximum dental benefit limits have not been raised since the inception and expansion of dental insurance in the 1970s. Of course, some plan limits are better than others. However, there has not been any appreciable increase (cost of living/inflation rate) in over 30 years. This has created the "crown-a-year club" whereby the patient will opt to wait for needed treatment in order to utilize the dental insurance. Many times, that opted decision ends up in more treatment and patient pain that could have been prevented if the yearly benefit level was reasonable. Dental insurance companies, in the interest of fairness and true support of the client's dental care needs, should make adjustments to the yearly maximum limit in benefits to reflect the current cost of living.

The insurance fee schedule should be fair and just to both the dentist and the patient. Patients often have access to the fee schedule and would correctly presume that the fee schedule lists those procedures that the dental insurance company provides benefits for. This is a true misrepresentation to the patient and creates a crack in the trusting doctor–patient relationship. The dentist must now explain to the patient his or her misinterpretation/misunderstanding of the policy that even though some procedures are listed, it does not mean it is covered. Meanwhile, the insurance company continues to promote its product. If the procedure is listed, it should be covered to prevent the many miscommunications that result from the described situation. If an insurance company wishes not to cover specific procedures, then it should not list those procedures on their fee schedules that represent covered benefit services. Likewise, once the yearly maximum limit on benefits has been reached, the dentist should not have to continue to accept the agreed-upon fee schedule because the insurance company no longer has to adhere to it. As mentioned previously, the insurance company adsorbs no more losses, but the dentist continues to adsorb the loss in reduced fees per the "take it or leave it" contract. In such a situation the insurance company is clearly taking advantage of the dentist. Again, some states have or are in the process of legislation to end such practices.

Due to the low insurance fees, many dentists are tempted to submit dental claims with inaccurate coding. By simply adding a surface or billing for a surgical extraction but only performing a routine extraction is committing fraud on state and federal levels.

True Case (3)

A large multistate corporate dental service organization (DSO) was asked by the federal government (Medicaid) to provide charts for 60 patients that had extractions. The DSO requested an outside dental consultant to review the charts, including radiographs, and the billing. It was found that the charts were written with all the same detail for a surgical extraction on all the extractions billed. Upon review of the accompanying radiographs, most (over 90%) were routine. Some root tips were in tissue. Fraud was committed.

True Case (Example) (4)

For every extraction the insurance is billed for a surgical extraction. The chart is written to support a surgical extraction was done. The X-ray however is questionable. Upon review by the insurance company, they find that it has been done for 12 years. The overpayment was $50.00 (for ease of discussion). The insurance company then does a retrospective audit:

Claimed incorrect/contested *fee* ($50)

×

Rate of code usage (40/week)

×

Number of years enrolled (12 = 524 weeks)

=

$1 048 000 DEMAND

Some dental insurance policies may dictate that dentists may not perform a covered procedure because the insurance company unilaterally decides it "is beyond the normal scope of the 'typical' general practitioner" [6]. The insurance company's decision to allow or disallow a proper referral to a specialist, when the general dentist finds it necessary, is an interference in the doctor–patient relationship. It interferes with the dentist's ability to seek the best care for their patient. It also forces unwanted issues with the ethical principles of autonomy and non-malfeasance as found in the ADA Code of Ethics.

As mentioned before, it may also force the dentist to perform treatment beyond their capabilities to accommodate the patient and find themselves in a risk management dilemma. There is also the rare situation where some insurance companies' policies may force a general dentist to attempt treatment beyond his or her capabilities when the guidelines make the general dentist financially liable for the services of a referred specialty treatment. In other words, "Services inappropriately referred may be determined to the financial responsibility of the Primary Care Dentist" [7]. Some insurance company policies will only pay "specialist fees" (molar root canals, periodontal surgery, extraction of impacted teeth) to a specialist and not to the general dentist even if he or she is more than capable to treat these situations. These are clearly intrusions into the doctor–patient relationship.

If the stakeholders (the patient, the doctor, the consultant, and the insurance company) work together and become knowledgeable in the policy benefits, become an advocate for the patient's autonomy, become vigilant in protecting the patient from ill-conceived practices, and become a truly caring benefit provider and respect the doctor–patient relationship, the patient will remain the focus of all the stakeholders. Hopefully, the issues raised will bring a better understanding so all stakeholders will work together in the interest of better dental health.

References

1 (a) ADA Survey (2016). Medicaid fee-for-service reimbursement rates for child and adult dental care services for all states. https://www.ada.org/~/media/ ADA/Science%20and%20Research/HPI/Files/HPIBrief_0417_1.pdf, p. 12 (accessed 26 November 2018) (b) ADA Health Policy Institute. Dental benefits coverage in the U.S. https://www.ada.org/~/media/ADA/Science%20and%20 Research/HPI/Files/HPIgraphic_1117_3.pdf?la=en

2 Consultant Guidelines, Reference Guide for Specialty Referrals, Managed DentalGuard Specialty Referral Department, Guardian Insurance Company, 2010.

3 Code of Ethics, American Association of Dental Consultants, 2010.

4 Graskemper, J. (June 2002). A new perspective on dental malpractice: Practice enhancement through risk management. *Journal of the American Dental Association* 133: 755.

5 Code of Ethics, American Dental Association, 2010.

6 Consultant Guidelines, Criteria for Reimbursement of Specialty Referrals, Blue Cross/Blue Shield, 2010.

7 Consultant Guidelines, Inappropriate Referrals, Aetna Advantage Plus Dental/ DMO, 2010.

2

Insurance Negotiations

> *Whether you think you can do a thing,*
> *or whether you think you can't do a thing,*
> *you're right.*
> **Henry Ford**

> *If the only tool you have is a hammer,*
> *you tend to see every problem as a nail.*
> **Abraham Maslow**

Dentists that started out from scratch or bought a practice may want to consider being a provider for some Preferred Provider Organization (PPO) insurances because it will generate some new patients into a new or existing practice. Existing practices that have found a downturn in new patients due to the economy may consider a dental insurance PPO agreement to be more accommodating to patients looking for a new dentist. There are basically three reasons for joining a PPO: 1) You do not have enough patients. 2) You are a new practice and looking for fast growth. 3) Patients are leaving the practice because you are not on their dental insurance panel of dentists from which they get a discounted fee. A good way to see if you need to join is to have your front office personnel make note of how many phone calls ask if you take their insurance. Of those phone calls, see how many have become patients over a three-month period. If there is a good percentage of the phone call inquiries not making appointments because you are not accepting their particular PPO, you might want to reconsider.

Once signing the PPO agreement, it will take some time because many businesses renew their insurance policies on a yearly basis. Even though your name is listed for an insurance company when you sign on, it may take a while for patients to realize that you are on the PPO list.

Signing a provider contract with a dental insurance company has many contractual issues and is beyond the scope of this book. Prior to signing any

Leadership and Communication in Dentistry, First Edition. Joseph P. Graskemper.
© 2019 John Wiley & Sons, Inc. Published 2019 by John Wiley & Sons, Inc.

contract, it is highly advisable to seek legal advice for proper understanding of the contract. One of the major issues is the fee schedule that you will be held to for payment of your services. It is usually 40–60% less than your UCR fee for your area and dependent on the insurance company; some are better than others. The fee schedule is negotiable in certain situations depending on the demographics of your area, your specialty or area of expertise, and the number of other dentists in your area that are already providers. The negotiation of the contract and/or fee schedule also depends on the insurance company policy. Some simply do not negotiate. With some time and a little hard work, you may find one or two insurance companies willing to negotiate an individual fee schedule. Remember only a two to five dollar increase on a procedure adds up over time. As time passes, the chances of negotiation are less and less as the insurance company gains a stronger presence in the dental market.

True Case (Example) (5)

If you charge $100 (for ease of discussion) for a one-surface restoration and negotiate a $5 raise in the fee schedule, that pays $60 for the restoration.

$5×10 (number of restorations per month) = $50 more per month

$50×52 weeks = $2600 more per year

$2600×2 years (till next possible negotiation) = $5200 more than you would have if you did not negotiate the fee schedule

If you can get that $5 raise on possibly four procedures, that would result in a $20 800 more income over the two years without doing anything more than a little time of asking for a better fee schedule.

In your negotiations you must develop your insurance profile. Your profile includes your strengths and your current Usual, Customary, and Reasonable (UCR) fees for your top 25 procedures. Among your strengths you should point out your location, the number of dentists in your area, and any specialty credential or certifications. Your location is very important since dentists in rural areas usually have a better chance at negotiating the insurance fee schedule since it is most likely there are less dentists on the insurance company PPO list when compared to a city environment. The number of dentists also is very important because the more dentists accepting a particular insurance plan, the less likely any negotiations are possible. Have one of your staff go online to see who in your area is on various insurance company PPO lists and then decide if the field is relatively still open or not. Your UCR fees should be at least at the 80–90th percentile. By giving the top 25 UCR fees in your practice, the insurance company will see the size of discount you must give to utilize their fee schedule. There are several fee comparison services available such as www.fairhealthconsumer.org or Henry Schein Digital Practice Analysis Tool (DPAT) fee analyzer. Remember you can always give a courtesy discount to non-insurance patients or even a pro bono case if the patient is in need of dental care and does not have the funds to cover 100% of your UCR.

When pursuing an affiliation with a certain PPO, be aware that many of the fee schedules that insurance companies use are shared and leased from each other. In other words, ABC Insurance Company may be using or leasing the fee schedule to XYZ Insurance Company. Per the contract you sign, you may be agreeing to honor other companies' fee schedule for those patients with that insurance. It is always necessary to have legal advice prior to signing any agreement/contract.

When contacting the insurance company, preferably by e-mail or certified letter (to maintain a credible "paper trail"), the person you need to contact is a recruiter or retention specialist. The professional relations person or agent is not the one to talk to because they do not have an equitable interest in you becoming or remaining a PPO provider. The recruiter or retention specialist usually has some interest, because they normally get some payment/bonus for having new dentists sign on or maintain dentists in a needed area. The vice president or other high-ranking administration person does not have much concern either, since they will be paid whether or not you sign on.

Once a staff member gets the right person to talk to and their e-mail or phone number, it is best to have the dentist make the contact with the recruiter/retention specialist rather than an auxiliary personnel. Most insurance personnel who deal at that level usually have past dental training as an assistant or receptionist and normally have respect for the dentist.

In your e-mail or letter, be sure to keep the expected response time short (two to three weeks) to maintain forward progression quickly so you can make a decision as soon as possible. If you get an insurance company to issue you a fee increase proposal based on your request, do not simply accept the first proposal. Request a review in a timely manner, stating that you were expecting a more respectable update fee. They may request you to pick five to seven procedure codes that you wish to further upgrade. Do a little homework and submit the information along with a reason for your deserving a better fee. You may also like to point out that your needed dental supplies to provide proper care for their clients and using quality materials have increased yearly by _____%, and such an increase is expected from the insurance company for the sake of continued proper care of their clients. All proposals should have the company's letterhead or logo to ensure validity of the offer whether it is via e-mail or postal service. Once you accept the offer, which may be valid for up to two years, get a start date and end date. A few months prior to your end date, you will need to renegotiate again. Try and do this yearly reevaluation of various plans in early fall. This allows you to consider renegotiating, if possible, the fee schedules prior to the year-end. This is the time many insurance companies decide to change or upgrade their fees and coincides with employers reviewing their health insurance policies for the coming year. It is the best time of the year to negotiate. Remember to do this yearly, because if you do not renegotiate, the insurance fees will possibly be automatically downgraded to their current insurance fee schedule. When you do your yearly negotiated update, be sure to use the fees that you will have in place in the coming year and not use the current year's UCR fees. Also, for a while after the new negotiated fee schedule is in place, have a staff member to double-check that the new insurance fee schedule that you agreed to actually is being honored by the insurance company's Predetermination or Pre-authorization and Explanation of Benefits (EOB) or Payment Detail.

In summary the seven steps to negotiate:

1) Build a profile.
2) Identify your leverage.
3) Get to the right person.
4) Write the letter.
5) Negotiate past the first proposal.
6) Written acceptance with insurance company logo.
7) Track, monitor, and set expiration date. (Ben Tuinei, personal emails: ben@everestadvocates.com)

Below are two sample letters that may be used. One pays more attention to the rural location of the practice. The other is more in-depth paying attention to the credentials of the dentist. Be sure to follow up if you do not receive a reply by the date stated in your letter. This follow-through shows you are committed serious about seeking a fairer fee schedule.

The Rural Practice

Negotiating Letter #1

(Date)

To Whom It May Concern (or the agent's name):

Dr. _____ has diligently served (insurance company) patients in this community and has the desire to continue providing the highest quality of dental care to patients who are dependent on (insurance company) for dental treatment. However, on account of the rural nature of the location in which the practice is located, the fees you assigned are unsustainable. We would like to request that our fees be reviewed and properly adjusted to reflect the true nature of the area in which we provide dental treatment. While we understand that all residents in our community are dependent on us for dental services, the current (insurance company) fees present a financial threat in allowing us to continue rendering dental services to those that need us.

We are requesting a fee schedule review and would like for you to consider following the same actuarial standards that all PPO plans follow in improving your fee schedule by at least 25%.

Please send your response within 2 weeks of the above date to me directly at: E-mail---- drsmile@happydental.com

Respectfully, (Ben Tuinei, personal email: Ben@everestadvocates.com)

Negotiating Letter #2

(Date)

To Whom It May Concern (or the agent's name):

Dear _____,

I have been given your e-mail address as being the retention specialist for (insurance company) in my region. Every year I must reevaluate my continuation in various dental insurance plans due to the ever-increasing (7–10%/year) cost of overhead (materials, staffing, office needs). I am writing to express concern and frustration with the current fee schedule you have assigned me. I've been a loyal provider of your PPO plan for several years and have provided great quality care to patients from your PPO network. I do enjoy providing dental treatment to all my patients and the feedback I get is that they enjoy having me as their dentist. I am writing you because the financial arrangement I have with you is interfering with the sustainability of this practice. The truth is, your assigned fee schedule is unsustainable and doesn't support the type of dentistry I deliver to your enrollees.

I would like to take this opportunity to request an increase in the (insurance company) PPO Fee Schedule. Good business means adequate profitability. You have a responsibility to your company to assure this, as do I to my company. It is in that spirit, as good business companies, that I would like to open a channel of communication with you regarding my services to your clients – my patients – and to begin negotiations for a benefit to us both.

I feel it is essential that you are familiar with who I am. I graduated from _____ University, attended _____ Graduate School, a dental degree from _____University in 1977 and a _____ certificate/ degree from _____ School of _____ in School Town, California, in 1987. (Tell about your self and what separates you or makes you different from other dentists. Tell about your self and what you do within your community and professionally outside your office. Maybe include some of your history that pertains. You are trying to get the person to get to know you.)

As you can see, I am not just an ordinary regular general dentist. I am very proficient and caring in my care for my patients and considered one of the top practices in my area. I am not a clinic with recent graduates as associates. I am the only dentist in my practice providing personal care for your clients. Bottom line, I am exactly the kind of practice that you want to market to employers.

I am aware that many insurers are being forced to follow the new Fair Health database in determining fair and reasonable charges to patients who seek medical and dental services from doctors outside of their PPO network. I have taken the time to compare my fees to those found on www.fairhealthconsumer. org. The UCR dental fees they list for my zip code are equal to or slightly greater than what I charge.

The fees currently offered through (insurance company) are 40–60% less than my typical fees and thus 40–60+% less than what Fair Health has listed as UCR for our area. As an out-of-network provider, (insurance company) would see claims from my practice that would reflect current UCR levels for fees in my area and thus be 40–60% higher than what you would be paying my practice. I am also sure that you understand my concerns regarding the contract clauses I previously mentioned and currently working on to address.

I suggest we meet in the middle and we use this third-party source for the fee schedule. I am willing to contract with (insurance company) as a preferred in network provider, if (insurance company) will agree to Fair Health UCR fees for my zip code less 20%. We are confident that you will see the advantage to this arrangement and the Win-Win business agreement it creates for both our companies.

Since this letter is to open the negotiation for this new business arrangement between (insurance company) and _____ DDS PLLC, I would like a response from you by (specific date). I look forward to this acknowledgment and an open communication between our companies that will provide each of us with the benefit the other can offer.

Sincerely, (Ben Tuinei, personal email: Ben@everestadvocates.com)

3

Preferred Provider Organization (PPO) Contractual Issues

Never let the fear of striking out get in your way.
Babe Ruth

Life is what happens to you when you're busy making other plans.
John Lennon

Being a dental provider for patients with dental insurance has some issues that you must be aware of: reduced fees (as discussed in Chapter 2), diagnosed treatment reviewed by the insurance company, Most Favored Nation (MFN) Clause (fee cap to lowest insurance fee schedule accepted), bundling of procedures, fee cap on non-covered services, downgrading or downcoding of treatment, coordination of benefits, delayed payment, nonpayment, limits on restoration replacements, limits on yearly treatment costs, and possible annual or biannual office visitation, to name a few, These are just a few of the more important contractual issues, and a complete discussion is beyond the scope of this chapter. When reviewing an insurance preferred provider contract, always seek proper legal advice regarding the impact on you and your practice.

In your initial dealings with a dental insurance company, you must understand that many procedures need to have predetermination via a treatment review of your proposed care for your patient. Whether or not you knowing it is covered, you must get used to verifying the patient's needs to a third party, possibly not even a dentist. If you decide to appeal a denial for proposed treatment, it is good to be adversarial in an educative manner and not to make it an argument. Take it on as to educate the other person to your insight of the needed treatment.

The MFN Clause simply states that there is a guarantee that the patient will receive terms at least as favorable as those provided to any other patient [1].

Leadership and Communication in Dentistry, First Edition. Joseph P. Graskemper.
© 2019 John Wiley & Sons, Inc. Published 2019 by John Wiley & Sons, Inc.

True Case (Example) (6)
You have signed on a Dental Insurance Company A's fee schedule, which has set a fee for a crown at $500. Although it is low, most of the people who live and work in the area have this insurance. You have tried not to get involved with dental insurance companies' PPOs but find it hard to sustain a profitable practice without it. Insurance Company B is trying to expand into the region by offering dentists a better fee schedule but also has an MFN Clause. Insurance Company B's fee schedule is better at $750 for a crown. You sign on to it hoping more new patients will be forthcoming and increase the practice's income. You submit for payment for a completed crown for your patient and their client and only receive 50% (the insurance company's portion) of $500 rather than the expected 50% of $750 with a note stating the MFN Clause in the contract you signed.

This allows the insurance company (if they find out that you accepted a lower fee for the same procedure and this is easy due to coordination of benefits clauses and the leasing/sharing of fee schedules) to pay less than the agreed-upon fee since you signed their contract containing an MFN Clause. You are now forced to accept the Dental Insurance Company A's lower fee schedule as the one fee schedule dictating what all the other insurance companies you have signed on to that have an MFN Clause will pay for a procedure.

MFN Clauses have been found to be upheld in most courts as legal in the interest of lowering healthcare costs even though the argument of being anticompetitive has been brought forth. It is best to negotiate this clause out of the contract.

Bundling of procedures is very common among PPO plans. The American Dental Association Current Dental Terminology Code book (CDT 2017: Dental Procedure Codes), which is updated yearly, actually supports the insurance companies' wanting to bundle various procedures: one code for a pin (D2951) and another for a core buildup including any pins (D2950) [2]. A very common and simple example of bundling of procedures with insurance companies, which is combining one to two procedures together for one, is the bundling pin placement with core buildups and then bundling core buildups with crowns for increased insurance profits. Rather than paying for each procedure individually, as is in this case, three procedures (pins, core buildup, and crown), the dentist is only paid an all-inclusive crown fee, which was the same as the crown individually. Hence you are doing the buildup and pin at no charge. Before the insurance companies' involvement in dentistry, there was no bundling. The expertise of placing a pin and a buildup including the cost of materials is entirely very different. Theoretically and ideally, treatment rendered should be unbundled and billed properly for every service rendered to be honest and fair to the provider and to the patient. It is important for the patient to know the quality and quantity of treatment provided. When it is all bundled together or all included, the patient does not realize that amount of treatment rendered because it is only the crown that they remember since that is all they see. Let the insurance company bundle it. Let us not do it to ourselves.

Fee capping for non-covered services has been found to be illegal in some states. This occurs when a procedure is not covered by the insurance company, but according to the terms of the PPO contract, you are only allowed to charge that which is on the fee schedule and not your Usual, Customary, and Reasonable (UCR) fee for the clients of that dental insurance company. Hence, in your need to provide certain procedures not covered by the patient's policy, you must still accept only the fee that is on his or her insurance company fee schedule as your full fee even though the insurance company does not pay their fair share of the fee.

There is also the common occurrence of the insurance company downgrading the code on their Estimation of Benefits (EOB) form. For example, you submit for a small two-surface composite restoration on a molar. The insurance company downgrades it to an amalgam restoration. The patient upon receipt of the insurance EOB now wants to change the restoration to amalgam due to cost. You can still do the composite restoration, but the patient must understand the additional cost incurred. Though not much, it places the dentist in a "selling" situation by which he or she must now explain or support their original diagnosis to place a composite rather than an amalgam. This can also be seen in the situation when the dentist submits for a crown on a molar and the predetermination is denied because the "dental consultant" decides that not enough tooth structure is missing to warrant a crown. Again, the dentist is in a challenging situation with the patient to reeducate the patient regarding the need for the crown. The patient, being cost-conscious, would rather go with what the "dental consultant" and insurance company are willing to pay. This can put a strain on the doctor–patient relationship. Hence, you must have good communication skills to lead the patient to the proper treatment regardless of insurance coverage.

Some dental benefit plans have "non-duplication of benefits" or "coordination of benefits" provisions. This means that the secondary plan will not pay any benefits if the primary plan paid the same or more than what the secondary plan allows for that procedure. If the primary insurance is less than the secondary insurance, the secondary insurance should pay the difference of the primary insurance payment and a higher secondary insurance fee unless, of course, the secondary has an MFN Clause as mentioned before.

True Case (Example) (7)

If both the primary and secondary carriers pay for the service at 80% level but the primary carrier allows $100 and the secondary carrier normally allows $80 for the same treatment, the secondary carrier would not make any additional payment. This is due to the secondary insurance company's belief that you have already been paid for the crown and you are not entitled to double payment even if both payments still do not cover your full UCR fee. However, if the primary carrier only pays 50% rather than 80% of the dentist's allowed fee of $100 ($50), then the secondary carrier would reduce its payment by the amount paid by the primary plan and pay the difference. In this case, the secondary carrier would pay $14 ($80×80% = $64 then minus $50 paid by the primary = $14).

When dealing with insurance companies, realize that you have a delay in payment as compared with non-insurance patients who normally pay at the time of treatment or agree to a payment plan. Insurance companies may take up to three months and maybe even longer to pay their portion of the agreed fee. Many states have laws like New York State's Prompt Payment Law, Insurance Law Section 3224-a, which establishes both time limits and sanctions for insurance companies delayed payment practices [3, 4]. This is of considerable importance in running a successful profitable practice. At first, it is a financial strain to continue providing patient care, but not being paid in a timely manner. Hence, it is paramount that the patient's portion of the balance due is collected at the time of service. After approximately three months, the cash flow will increase and balance out such that the patients you are treating currently will be paying their patient portion and you will be receiving the insurance balance due for previous patients' treatment. Many of the delays in treatment are caused by the insurance company's need for more information, misrecorded patient identification (group number, social security number, wrong address, etc.), or simply lost paperwork/e-claim. Submitting to insurance companies should be electronically done to improve the speed of communications.

In rare situations, an insurance company will deny payment even after issuing an EOB that stated treatment is within the policy and payment will be made upon completion of the treatment as submitted on the predetermination. The insurance company will then point out on the payment of benefits form that the EOB is not a guarantee of payment and based upon their "dental consultant's" review, payment will not be made. This type of situation should be appealed because you and the patient have detrimentally relied on the EOB for proper payment under the policy. The patient should also get involved and contact the state's insurance department (see True Case (1)).

Dental insurance company policies place a time limit on the replacement of prosthodontic and certain other procedures. It may range from 5 to 10 years that must elapse between replacing a crown, partial or full denture. Orthodontically it may be just a once-in-a-lifetime coverage. These limitations on benefits for a certain amount of time are generally held to by the insurance company as non-negotiable.

There is also a maximum yearly limit on the amount the insurance company will pay. This maximum limit may be from $1000 to $2500 per year, and in rare exceptions this may be unlimited. In the 1970s, a $1000 per year was reasonable coverage to provide most of the patient's needed care. Over 40 years later with no change in the yearly maximum, it does not provide the same coverage. Therefore, patients and dentists must properly sequence treatment to work within this yearly limitation. Many times, due to the patient's needs, this is not possible. However, the patient states they do not want to or is unable to go over that yearly limit. This often results in more treatment than would have been necessary if the patient were treated in a timely manner. The simple filling has now turned into a root canal while waiting for the next year benefit limits to begin again. What has been created is the "crown-a-year club" as mentioned in Chapter 1. Many times, the sequencing of treatment may take place over two to three years to complete the needed dental care while maintaining the patient's dental health such that it does not deteriorate during that time period. Hence, proper patient education through co-diagnosis is essential [5]. It should also be noted that most PPOs have a deductible that must be met by the patient before any insurance payments are made.

Oftentimes, the patient wants to complete their treatment in a more timely manner. Then they ask if you would honor the insurance fee that was allowed on their other work that was within the yearly benefit level to be helpful in their completing their treatment. The dentist is now in a situation trying to explain that the crown will now cost twice as much as the crown done last month under the yearly maximum benefit level. Many dentists will simply accept the full insurance fee from the patient. This avoids the wrong patient impression of the dentist only caring about the money and not the patient.

When dealing with various insurance company PPOs, there may be a clause in the contract allowing an insurance company representative to make an annual office visitation. Normally a representative from the insurance company will call and make an appointment to visit the dental office. This is done so they can be reassured that you are following proper dental practice regulations (Occupational Safety and Health Administration [OSHA], Health Insurance Portability and Accountability Act [HIPAA], universal precautions, sterilization, etc.) for the protection of their clients. It is normally a short, nonintrusive visit. However, you must take the lead to control the visit. First and foremost, it should not be a fishing expedition by the representative.

When setting the appointment time for the in-office review, make it at a time when there are no patients in the office and request which clients' charts they wish to review. They are only allowed to review those patients that are clients of the insurance company and not have access to all patient charts. You should also make a request per HIPAA that the representative have a signed patient authorization to review the chart. This is normally already given by the patient at the time of signing onto the insurance plan. Nevertheless, make sure all the paperwork is proper. These visits normally do not take long, and the representative is normally understanding of the intrusion they cause.

In recent advances in dental insurance provider agreements, insurance companies have placed themselves, through a rating system, in a position to direct patients to dentists of their choosing based on tiering of their contracted providers. To simply ignore these advances and not accept insurance is not a realistic decision for most dentists, especially the newly graduated dentist with an average school debt of over $200 000. According to the American Dental Education Association (ADEA) 2017 survey, the average debt per graduating senior is $287 331 [6].

Insurance companies are attempting to rate their dental panel providers, usually through a subsidiary or contracted third party. They present this *opportunity* for the dentists as a way to make patients *engaged consumers* of services. This is a very real problem in presenting dental services as a commodity that transforms dentists into sellers of services and/or merchants that an *engaged consumer* can shop for from a list of insurance company self-interest rated providers. They inform their panel of dentists that this is a better *interactive patient–provider communication platform*. However, they do not mention that they have control of that communication through their rating system – not the dentist – not the patient. It is also pointed out by the insurance company that they are not going to charge the dentist for this rating system and that it is *offered as a courtesy for your relationship* with the insurance company [7].

To facilitate this new intrusion, insurance companies will not issue a new updated fee schedule without the dentist's signed acceptance of this new addendum to the provider agreement. This new addendum may read, "In addition, (insurance company) reserves the right to direct Participants to selected dentist and/or influence a Participant's choice of dentist. This may include, but is not limited to, the segmentation or tiering of the dental network" [7]. These clauses are not only found in the contract or addendum but may be referred to as being in the insurance company policy manual that you must abide by. Therefore, with this clause, the insurance company could even call your patient who is one of their clients and redirect them out of your office and into another dental office.

Another intrusion that is highly questionable ethically is the new clauses showing up in the agreements and policy manuals that disallows treatment. This clause is a very clear intrusion into the doctor–patient relationship and patient autonomy by not allowing the dentist to provide the procedure that was disallowed even if the patient and doctor mutually agree to the needed procedure. A disallow clause not only eliminates any possible insurance benefit payment but also prohibits the dentist from charging or accepting any money from the patient. Under this new system, the patients and dentists become entirely subservient to the insurance company's want for profits. Prohibition of collection for needed treatment rendered to informed and consented patients even when the insurance company does not cover it is also seen in clauses that refer to the possible future bankruptcy of the insurance company [7]. There should be a clause included in the agreement that the dentist will be notified of any changes to the provider policy manual.

Hold harmless clauses that relieve the insurance company of any liability arising from the dentist, and the dentist will reimburse the insurance company for any loses that the insurance company may have due to the dentist. These types of clauses are very typical of various contracts to protect each party. It is best to have a mutual hold harmless for both the dentist and the insurance company.

Audit payback clause allows the insurance company to reduce future payments to the dentist based on any insurance overpayment or mistaken payments per the insurance company audits. Within this clause should be a notification of such an audit, amount due, claim information, and a time limit to "claw back" their mistaken payment.

Shared plans clause allows the insurance company to have other insurance providers to have access to their dental insurance plan including the fee schedule and make the dentist agree to those other plans by being affiliated with the original insurance company. With the current increase in mergers and acquisitions, there should be a clause regarding the notification of the dentist and whether he or she agrees to it or to opt out.

Some provider agreements state that the dentist must participate with all the plans the insurance company offers or not participate at all. Be very careful of these types of clauses because plans change and get dropped and added on yearly. The dentist may see five fee schedules, of which only one is financially feasible. The dentist then signs on thinking most of the new patients will have the good fee schedule only to find out that no one is on that plan except those clients that are out of state or after one year the good fee schedule has been dropped and the patients are now all on the lower fee schedules. There should be 90-day notification to the dentist that the insurance company is dropping or changing a fee schedule.

There are many more considerations in signing a provider agreement such that you must seek proper local legal and practice management advice prior to signing any such agreement.

References

1 Thomson Reuters Practical Law, Glossary, Most Favored Nations Provisions, 2018. https://content.next.westlaw.com/Document/I0f9fe70bef0811e28578f7cc c38dcbee/View/FullText.html?contextData=(sc.Default)&transitionType=Default (accessed 9 June 2018).

2 American Dental Association Current Dental Terminology Code Book (CDT 2017: Dental Procedure Codes), p. 24.

3 New York State Law, Section 3224 Insurance Law, September 1997. https://www.dfs.ny.gov/insurance/circltr/2000/cl00_06.htm (accessed 8 December 2018).

4 New York State, Office of General Counsel, Department of Finance, 5 May 2011. https://www.dfs.ny.gov/insurance/ogco2011/rg110503.htm (accessed 9 June 2018).

5 Graskemper, J. (2011). *Professional Responsibility in Dentistry: A Practical Guide to Law and Ethics*, 167. Ames, IA: Wiley-Blackwell.

6 American Dental Education Association Survey. https://www.adea.org/ GoDental/Money_Matters/Educational_Debt.aspx (accessed 8 December 2018).

7 Graskemper, J. (2018). The collapse of the doctor-patient relationship due to insurance company intrusions. *Journal of Dental Humanities* 2 (1/2, Winter/ Spring): 6.

4

Estimation of Benefits Problems

Can't always get what you want, but you get what you need.
Rolling Stones

Success is going from failure to failure without losing enthusiasm.
Winston Churchill

To treat patients legally and ethically within the standard of care and be a participating dental insurance provider, dentists must learn to properly communicate with the insurance companies for the benefit of their patients and the survival of their dental offices. The need for many procedures is routinely questioned by the insurance companies, such as crowns, buildups, scale and root planing with the placement of a locally delivered antibiotic, or replacing a missing tooth. Because the insurance company must verify the patient's needs, a predetermination is often needed. All predeterminations should be submitted with the dentist's full Usual, Customary, and Reasonable (UCR) fee. By doing so, the insurance company will make note of the UCR fees of all the submitting panel dentists to help determine their future fee schedule updates, if and when they do so. If you submit a predetermination with the insurance fee, it gives the insurance company the impression that your UCR fee is the same – hence a false UCR fee. The insurance company will see no need to improve its fee schedule based on your false UCR fee, which appears to be the same as on the insurance fee schedule. This brings down the insurance company's composite fee, which is based on submitted fees, and gives them reason to not raise their fee schedules.

Always use proper billing codes when submitting for payment to avoid delays in receiving an Estimation of Benefits (EOB) or payment. One of the most miscoded procedures is operative restorations. To prevent miscommunication regarding the surfaces of a restorative filling, the following guidelines might be helpful.

Rather than relying on your individual feeling or personal ethical conscience as to what is a fair basis for diagnosing and coding the size of operative restorations and as to when a restoration extends into another surface, a guide, upon which all can rely on for fair and equitable patient care, that outlines in a mutually fair and consistent manner, the correct diagnosis and coding for the number of surfaces actually restored is needed. For example, many class II restorations may extend more facially or lingually past the marginal ridge area. Without established guidelines, dentists are left to arbitrarily decide whether to include the extended portion as another surface, and the insurance companies, of course, would rather pay only for two surfaces when the restoration actually involves three. The real question arises when a traditional class II restorative preparation extends well into the facial or lingual area, thereby involving another surface. This can also be noted in large anterior restorations and large class V restorations that wrap around to other surfaces [1].

For proper diagnosis, treatment, and payment of services, each tooth is divided into four planes (two mesial-distally and two buccal-lingually), leaving nine surface areas as seen in Figure 4.1. Draw a line occlusally and create a plane mesial-distally 1 mm lingually from the lingual edge of the mesial and distal contacts. Likewise, draw a second line/plane through the occlusal surface 1 mm buccally of the contacts. These planes should approximate the cusps of a molar 1–2 mm toward the center of the occlusal center or the width of the incisal edge of the anterior teeth. See Figure 4.2. Similarly, draw a line buccal-lingually 1–2 mm of the marginal ridge for a posterior tooth

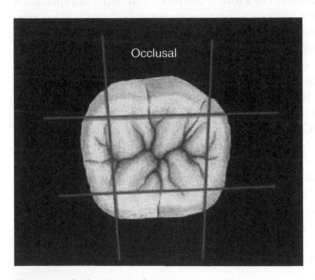

Figure 4.1 Occlusal view of a molar. *Source:* [1]. Reproduced with permission of *Dental Economics.*

Figure 4.2 Incisal view of an incisor. *Source:* [1]. Reproduced with permission of *Dental Economics.*

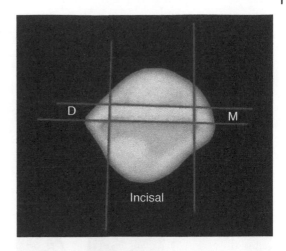

and the contact for an anterior tooth, sectioning the tooth into thirds. This should be approximately through the cusps of a molar 1–2 mm from the cusp tips from the marginal ridge. Or you can divide an anterior tooth 1–2 mm from the mesial and distal incisal angles, cutting the tooth into thirds mesial-distally and creating nine sections of a tooth. The planes should extend through the labial/buccal and lingual surfaces as shown in Figures 4.3 and 4.4 [1].

The illustrations show that as the tooth preparation extends into another plane, an added surface is encountered. As you prepare occlusally, mesially, or distally through the mesial or distal occlusal plane, another surface is encountered due to the undermining of the marginal ridges or the incisal corners for anterior teeth, which results in the need to restore another surface. Likewise, as you go buccally or lingually, you either undermine a cusp or are well beyond merely breaking the mesial or

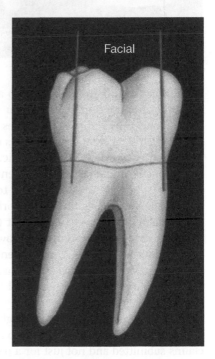

Figure 4.3 Buccal view of a molar. *Source:* [1]. Reproduced with permission of *Dental Economics.*

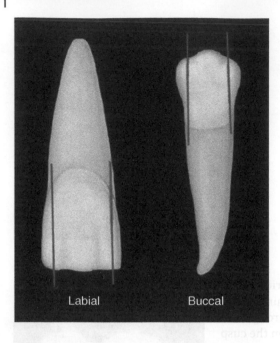

Figure 4.4 Facial view of an incisor and bicuspid. *Source:* [1]. Reproduced with permission of *Dental Economics.*

Labial   Buccal

distal contact and are actually into another surface. When preparing a large, deep facial abfraction/erosion, you would also encounter the mesial and/or distal plane; thus additional surfaces would require restoration [1].

The insurance company also uses coding information to compare your billing patterns to other dental practices on their panel. This is done to detect unreasonable and possibly fraudulent claims. Do not upgrade a procedure to a better paying code with the intent to receive a better payment. This is called upcoding. Many laws like New York's Penal Code Law 177 and the Federal False Claims Act look to the intent to defraud the insurance company or the Medicare/Medicaid systems by knowingly and willfully provide false information or omit information for payment [2, 3]. The Affordable Care Act removes the need to show intent to enforce a finding of fraud [4]. It only needs to show the possibility of a belief that fraud has occurred. Hence, a finding of fraud is much easier.

In a pattern of unnecessary, wrongly upcoded, or excessive claims for a certain procedure, you may be submitted to a full practice review. This is a review of all claims submitted and not just for a particular patient or procedure. Examples of fraudulent behavior would be waiving of the patient's co-payment, giving a discount to the patient and not to the insurance company, billing for extra surfaces for restorations, substituting the proper code with a better paying code, and billing for a crown when only an onlay was done.

If you have been profiled by the insurance company or Medicare/Medicaid systems, you need to involve the patient to verify the treatment was rendered.

You need to seek proper professionals to help answer such questioning. You want to reach a conclusion as soon as possible and, of course, end the cited behavior. They do not need to show you intended to defraud but only show in their belief that fraud has possibility occurred.

True Case (Example) (8)

For every occlusal filling on a maxillary first molar, the dentist submitted an occlusal–lingual for payment of an additional surface, or under every filling the dentist does, he or she also places a base or pulp cap (Dycal) and submits for it in addition to the filling. The dentist has been doing this for the past 12 years. The insurance company states that it is over-treatment and/or fraudulent billing. The insurance company may want to do an audit. A retrospective audit could be done to determine the amount owed due to a finding of fraudulent billing practices. Such an audit showing a small billing error, which they believe is fraud, may become very expensive. For ease of discussion, the claimed overpayment of just $2.00 for a procedure (adding a surface to an amalgam restoration) that is done 40 times a week for the 10 years you have been on the insurance company's panel would equal a demand of $41 600! ($2 × 40/ week × 520 weeks = $41 600).

Predeterminations are normally needed for any fixed or removable prosthodontics (crowns, bridges, implants, full and partial dentures). A predetermination is not needed for emergency treatment. There are some patients that will request an exact out-of-pocket cost even for a small restorative procedure. It is best advised to predetermine in such cases to prevent any misinformation to the patient that would alter their informed consent. It should be suggested to the patient that a predetermination be sent to see how much a contribution to their dental care the insurance company wishes to make toward their receiving needed care. Such a patient may even become upset if they end up paying more than expected because he or she was misquoted their patient portion. To provide the needed information for an EOB approval is paramount in obtaining the needed coverage for your patient needs and for you to get paid. With most predeterminations appropriate radiographs must also be submitted. Sometimes an intraoral photograph must also be provided to show that which is not easily seen on a radiograph image. To prevent most delays, provide the insurance company all the needed information (good diagnostic radiographs/ intraoral photographs) to allow benefits, and a short (one to two lines) descriptive phrase with the radiograph and photo (if needed) is all that is usually required for a positive EOB for you and your patient. This sounds like a lot of information to pass onto the insurance company, but once you have a system down, it is relatively easy. Most times it prevents further letter writing to convince the insurance company and help them understand your patient's needs.

True Case (9)

Upon receipt of a denial for a new crown that needed to be replaced because of marginal decay, the dentist being an advocate for the patient must verify the need. The caries was very noticeable on both the bitewing and periapical images and was beyond the replacement limits of the policy for prosthodontic replacements. The dentist took a periodontal probe placed in the cavitation at the margin showing a 2 mm depth and took a photo of it. He wrote an appeal letter and sent the photo to get an appealed approval. Although it took a couple of extra minutes to take the intraoral photo, by being an advocate for his patient, he also increased his production and the patient is now a multiple referrer to his practice.

Some examples of phrases are as follows:

Needed crown

Large alloy/composite undermining _____cusp/incisal edge is leaking and defective with decay.

_____ cusp/incisal edge fractured

Vertical explorable fracture line on _____ of tooth (see photo)

Tooth has had root canal therapy (RCT)

To correct super-eruption, prevent further collapse of the Mandibular/ Maxillary arch, and maintain the occlusal table so a bridge may be properly fabricated on the opposing arch

Buildup

_____cusp undermined by large defective alloy/composite

Due to RCT

In the case when the buildup is bundled, then there is no need to explain the need. However, when the buildup is not bundled with the crown and has been denied, take a radiograph or even an intraoral photograph after all caries has been removed and before you place the buildup to show the need. I have found that most insurance companies will cover the cost of a radiograph but not the intraoral photograph. Therefore, if the patient is overly concerned about out-of-pocket costs, a radiograph before and after the buildup is placed should suffice.

Bridge

All retainer/abutment teeth should have their individual need for the crown if possible.

To replace #_____ which has been missing for _____years, prevent further collapse of the occlusal table and to maintain the integrity of the _____arch

Night guard/bruxism appliance

Severe wear and attrition of incisal edges of anterior teeth due to severe bruxism, causing chipping of teeth #_____

Severe bruxism causing mobility of anterior teeth

Temporomandibular joint splint

Bilateral Temporomandibular Joint (TMJ) pain upon palpation, ___ (appropriate muscle) _____ extremely tender upon palpation, limited opening of _____mm, deviation of _____mm on opening, limited extrusion of _____mm and headaches_____ (AM/PM).

Sleep apnea device

Most insurance companies will not provide benefits for a sleep apnea device without a copy of the patient's Sleep Deprivation Report. This report is generated at a sleep center per the patient's physician. Depending on your state's laws, sleep deprivation study may only be requested by a physician. Hence, the easiest way to provide a sleep apnea device is to have the patient request their physician to order a sleep deprivation study and have a copy sent to you.

Scaling and root planing with intra-sulcular medication

Send copy of full mouth radiographs and a periodontal chart with probing depths. I have found the level of coverage varies greatly among the dental insurance companies. Some will provide benefits for sulcular pockets of 5 mm or greater, while some will not provide any benefit unless the sulcular pockets are 7 mm or greater. It also varies greatly on the threshold of severity as to whether they will cover intra-sulcular medications. Hence, the more information the better. If the pockets are not within the range to qualify for insurance benefits, you may be able to do a gross debridement and then a prophy, if there is calculus evident on the radiographs. Be specific as to whether you are doing code D4342, 1–3 teeth, or code D4341 for quadrant. Also, code D4346, scaling in presence of generalized moderate or severe gingival inflammation, may be used for those patients who have supra-bony pockets due to tissue inflammation [5].

True Case (10)

A dentist consistently diagnosed and coded all scaling and root planing as quadrants. The insurance company questioned and requested verification of 60 patients, all billed for 4 quadrants of scaling and root planing. It was found that most of the patients did not have more than three teeth with periodontal pocketing greater than 3 mm. Many patients did not even have periodontal charting done. A financial "claw-back" was made due to the audit and charges of fraud were made.

References

1 Graskemper, J. (1 June 2017). Surfaces for operative restorations: A guideline for diagnosis and proper billing. *Dental Economics* 107 (6): 30–32.

2 New York State Law, Penal Law, Article 177, Secrtion 177.00. http://ypdcrime.com/penal.law/article177.htm (accessed 10 June 2018).

3 U.S. Code Title 31, Subtitle III Chapter 37, Subchapter III Section False Claims. https://www.law.cornell.edu/uscode/text/31/3729 (accessed 10 June 2018).

4 Stevens and Lee, Summary of Fraud and Abuse Provisions of the Patient Protection and Affordable Care Act, April 22, 2010. http://www.stevenslee.com/summary-of-fraud-and-abuse-provisions-of-the-patient-protection-and-affordable-care-act (accessed 10 June 2018).

5 American Dental Association Current Dental Terminology Code Book (CDT 2017: Dental Procedure Codes), p. 39.

5

Appeals Letters

There are only two ways to live your life.
One is as though nothing is a miracle.
The other is as though everything is a miracle.
Albert Einstein

Do or not do.
There is no try.
Jedi Master Yoda

Even though you have provided the insurance company all the required information regarding the patient's needed dental care for proper benefit coverage, they may still refuse to provide benefits or alter the treatment plan per the insurance policy guidelines to the Least Costly Alternative Treatment (LCAT). Remember and be mindful that most predeterminations are reviewed not by a licensed dentist but by an administrative staff who are given mere guidelines on what to allow and what not to allow. Therefore, the first denial of your recommended treatment plan, being reviewed by a non-dentist, should be appealed and be reconsidered by the insurance company dental consultant.

The patient still needs to be informed of all options to maintain patient autonomy and a proper informed consent. A denial of insurance coverage should be based on one of the following reasons: 1) not a covered service under the policy, exceeds the yearly maximum, or does not meet the wait time for replacement or retreatment, 2) improper or missing documentation, and 3) a less costly alternative treatment per the policy. If you care to become more of an advocate for your patient to receive the needed dental care and to provide a healthy production level for your practice, you can write a letter appealing their decision to deny benefits. With just a little practice and using the following letter formats, you can easily request an appeal. Once you have built a library of letters for different situations, it becomes very easy. With minor changes regarding the specific patient, each letter is easily customized or adapted to that patient's need.

Leadership and Communication in Dentistry, First Edition. Joseph P. Graskemper.
© 2019 John Wiley & Sons, Inc. Published 2019 by John Wiley & Sons, Inc.

I personally believe that if you decide to accept dental insurance into your practice, you have an ethical responsibility to be an advocate for your patient. To sign up for insurance plans only to tell the patient it is not covered with the intent to collect your Usual, Customary, and Reasonable (UCR) fee in full is misleading to the patient and questionably unethical because the patient has partially based their decision to become your patient on your representation that you accept their insurance. This type of business format is misleading and questionably unethical.

Each of these situations requires a different letter to establish the insurance companies' need to review their denials and make proper benefit payment. Although each letter addresses a specific situation, there are some common threads running through most of them. It is suggested to cc a copy of the letter to the patient so they can see your adversarial efforts in obtaining proper dental insurance coverage. The patient will feel you care about them and their needs and will truly appreciate you and your office's extra effort. It becomes a practice builder.

Bundling of Core Buildup with the Crown

A prime example of bundling is the incorporation of the fee for a core buildup into the fee for a crown. By bundling procedures, the insurance company clearly makes more money by not paying for it, and you the dentist now are put in a standard of care situation and ethical decision of whether to pay for the materials for the buildup themselves or try to get by without the buildup. If needed, take a radiograph after the tooth is prepared but before the buildup is placed, thus showing the need for the buildup. You still may not get paid for it per your contract and forced to abide by the fee schedule that you agreed to. You may also take another radiograph, if you are so inclined, after the buildup is placed to show that is had been done.

To Whom It May Concern:
Please reconsider your denial of benefits for a core buildup for tooth #_____ for your client _____. According to the American Dental Association (ADA) Current Dental Terminology (CDT) code D2950, core buildup is not part of code D2750. Please see a copy of the ADA CDT enclosed as the set standard in the dental insurance Industry [1]. Please be aware that the ADA Council on Dental Benefit Programs has successfully challenged such insurance company policies. Also enclosed are two radiographs of pre- and post-placement of the core buildup.

To not provide coverage for these procedures would be a disservice to my patient and your client. To not allow benefits could be taken as Bad Faith Coverage and would have to be reported to the _____ State Department of

Insurance. To diagnose a patient's or client's dental needs without an examination is below the standard of care.

Thank you for your immediate cooperation in correcting the improper bundling of procedures and providing proper benefits for your client _____.

Sincerely,

New Crown Due to Marginal Caries

When a new crown is needed due to marginal decay and has already been submitted to the insurance company for an Estimation of Benefits (EOB) and denied because their review had determined that replacement is not needed because the need is not seen on the radiographs sent with the predetermination, a letter is then needed to express the need. If the decay is substantial, take an intraoral photo with an explorer or periodontal probe going into the carious margin. You can also circle the carious area on the photograph. This photo should be sent with the following letter.

Dear Dental Consultant,
(Sorry for no name, but you did not give me the courtesy of your name)

I truly understand the difficulty of screening insurance claim forms without seeing the patient. So, I am resubmitting because I believe in the patient's need.

My patient and your client, _____, is in need of replacing an old (over _____ years) crown on #_____ due to decay on the _____ margin as can be clearly seen in the bitewing radiograph. A periapical radiograph is also enclosed to show root canal therapy completed (if applicable). An intraoral photograph is attached showing the need to replace the crown (if needed).

Also, dental consultants should abide by the American Association of Dental Consultants Code of Ethics (AADC). The duties owed to the patient according to the AADC Code of Ethics may be found at "3E. All dental consultants should abide by the American Dental Association Code of Ethics." And as stated in Principle 4, "4B. The ethical aspects of dental consultant duties must always take precedence over economic aspects. 4C. The doctor-patient relationship, even indirect, is fiduciary, and must take precedence over economic or personal influences. 4D. The dental consultant must regard 'standard of care' the same for all providers" [2].

To not provide coverage for these procedures would be a disservice to my patient and your client. According to the standard of care in dentistry, reasonable care and diligence includes patient examination. To diagnose a patient's or client's dental needs without an examination is below the standard of care per se. To not replace these crowns would be dental care below the standard of care.

Failure to allow benefits for needed treatment would be taken as Bad Faith Coverage and would have to be reported to the _____ State Department of Insurance.

I understand that at times it is hard to determine benefits without seeing the patient. However, to not provide coverage for these procedures would be a disservice to my patient and your client.

Thank you for your immediate attention and providing proper care for your client and my patient, _____.

Sincerely,

Vertical Fracture Line

Many times a patient may exhibit a tooth with a vertical fracture line that requires a full coverage crown to prevent further fracturing and possible loss of tooth. Normally vertical fracture lines are not noticeable on the radiograph, and an intraoral photo should be taken to show the actual fracture line.

To Whom It May Concern:

Please reevaluate your denial of benefits for my patient and your client _____. Both teeth #_____ and #_____ have vertical, explorable fracture lines as can be seen in the attached intraoral photograph. This was originally reported on the initial predetermination.

I understand that at times it is hard to determine benefits without seeing the patient. However, to not provide coverage for these procedures would be a disservice to my patient and your client.

Both teeth are in need of full coverage crowns to prevent fracture of the tooth rendering it non-restorable. I can actually place my explorer into the fracture line on both teeth. (If applicable) Upon total removal of the failed alloy that undermines the lingual wall and covers the buccal cusps of #_____ and undermines the lingual wall of #_____, buildups will be needed to be done to properly prepare the tooth for full coverage crowns. Failure to do so will lead to premature failure of the crowns due to lack of proper support.

To not provide coverage for these procedures would be a disservice to my patient and your client. To not allow benefits could be taken as Bad Faith Coverage and would have to be reported to the _____ State Department of Insurance. To diagnose a patient's or client's dental needs without an examination is below the standard of care.

Also, you should be aware that dental consultants should abide by the American Association of Dental Consultants Code of Ethics. As stated in Principle 4, "4B. The ethical aspects of dental consultant duties must always take precedence over economic aspects. 4C. The doctor-patient relationship, even indirect, is fiduciary and must take precedence over economic or personal influences" [2].

Thank you for your cooperation in providing proper dental health care for your client.

Sincerely,

Substituting a Large Amalgam for a Survey Crown

Many times the insurance company will downgrade your treatment plan under the policy guideline of only allowing the "LCAT." A good example is the substitution of a planned full coverage crown for an abutment tooth for a partial denture. The tooth having a very large leaking/defective amalgam/composite overlaying or undermining a cusp where a clasp or rest seat would exert forces would be better served with a survey crown than another large amalgam/composite restoration.

To Whom It May Concern:

Tooth #_____ needs a full coverage crown. As can be seen in the enclosed radiograph, the decay completely undermines the cusp, and tooth #_____ has a completed root canal (if applicable).

To not place a full coverage crown and place a compromised amalgam filling will only lead to early breakdown, especially because a _____ partial denture will be clasping and resting on tooth #_____, making it an abutment/supporting essential tooth needed for proper fabrication, retention, and success of the _____ partial denture. Due to the entire cusp and total distal-facial aspect of the tooth being in amalgam, amalgam would not be the material of choice and lend itself to a questionable longevity of the restoration and the long-term success of the partial denture.

To not allow benefits for a full coverage crown would be a disservice to your client and my patient, _____. I am sure you want successful, predictable, and proper dental care for your client.

The crowns on teeth #_____ and _____ and the _____ partial denture have already been completed in the interest of the patient's dental health. (Some patients have a primary and a secondary insurance.) His primary dental insurance has already paid for these procedures (EOB enclosed).

Thank you for your immediate cooperation in providing proper benefits for needed dental care for you client and my patient _____.

Sincerely,

A Partial Denture Instead of Bridges

Insurance companies, in their best interests, may deny bridges to replace a missing tooth or teeth and recommend a partial denture. The LCAT Clause that is found in most if not all provider contracts allows for the insurance company to only pay for the least costly treatment, not the ideal or what the doctor and patient agree is the best treatment for the patient's needs.

To Whom It May Concern:

Please reevaluate your denial of proper dental benefits for your client, _____. To force a patient to wear a partial denture for only one tooth is not only unreasonable but seems punitive when proposed by the patient's insurance company. Honoring the patient's autonomy and a trusting doctor–patient relationship, the best alternative to replace only one tooth is an implant. A bridge from _____ is also acceptable in this situation. I must point out that your client has had a bridge from _____ for over ___ years and needs replacement due to caries on the buccal of ____. The only explanation for your denial is to increase profits with total disregard to proper patient care, which I consider unethical.

Also, dental consultants should abide by the American Association of Dental Consultants Code of Ethics. The duties owed to the patient according to the AADC Code of Ethics may be found at "3E. All dental consultants should abide by the American Dental Association Code of Ethics." And as stated in Principle 4, "4B. The ethical aspects of dental consultant duties must always take precedence over economic aspects. 4C. The doctor-patient relationship, even indirect, is fiduciary and must take precedence over economic or personal influences. 4D. The dental consultant must regard 'standard of care' the same for all providers" [2].

I understand that at times it is hard to determine benefits without seeing the patient. It should be pointed out that to diagnose treatment without seeing the patient is considered below the standard of care and malpractice. To not allow benefits for a fixed bridge would be a true disservice and possibly be taken as Bad Faith Coverage, whereby I would have to refer your client to the State Department of Insurance.

Thank you for your immediate attention and cooperation in providing proper dental care for your client and my patient, _____.

Sincerely,

Disallow Prophylaxis After Scale and Root Planing

In the insurance company's interest, it is not uncommon that the insurance company may want to bundle or include the prophylaxis appointment into the scale and root planing appointment.

To Whom It May Concern:

Please reconsider your denial of benefits for your client, _____.

A prophylaxis is NOT part of another procedure. If it is done as part of another procedure, it would not have a separate ADA Procedure Code.

Nowhere in your contract or your fee schedule is it stated that it is contained in another procedure.

D1110 is described as "Prophylaxis for Adult." There is no mention in the ADA CDT of D1110 being included with any other procedure [3].

D4341 is described as "Periodontal scaling and root planning – four or more teeth per quadrant." There is no mention of a prophylaxis being included in the ADA CDT [4].

Also dental consultants should abide by the American Association of Dental Consultants Code of Ethics. The duties owed to the patient according to the AADC Code of Ethics may be found at "3E. All dental consultants should abide by the American Dental Association Code of Ethics." This includes abiding to the ADA CDT codes. And as stated in Principle 4, "4B. The ethical aspects of dental consultant duties must always take precedence over economic aspects. 4C. The doctor-patient relationship, even indirect, is fiduciary and must take precedence over economic or personal influences. 4D. The dental consultant must regard 'standard of care' the same for all providers" [2].

Any further delay in payment for treatment rendered to your client will be taken as Bad Faith Coverage and will be reported to the _____ State Department of Insurance.

Thank you in allowing proper benefits for your client, _____.

Sincerely,

Sometimes a Predetermination Is Sent Back Stating that the Radiograph Is Not Readable or Does Not Show the Entire Tooth, When in Fact the Opposite is True

To Whom It May Concern:
I do not know who reviewed this radiograph but it was obviously not a dentist. Please understand that I know how difficult it is to confirm needed treatment without even seeing the patient. However, as can be seen, and I circled #_____ so you may see it more clearly that the entire tooth is present on the radiograph. The _____ is in need of replacement due to decay on the _____ margin. If you took the time to examine the patient with proper instruments (a mirror, explorer, and periodontal probe, you would find the decay present as stated; of course, that would depend on your diagnostic skills and experience). An intraoral photo, if needed, is also attached for your benefit.

Dental consultants should abide by the American Association of Dental Consultants Code of Ethics. The duties owed to the patient according to the AADC Code of Ethics may be found at "3E. All dental consultants should abide by the American Dental Association Code of Ethics." And as stated in

Principle 4, "4B. The ethical aspects of dental consultant duties must always take precedence over the economic aspects. 4C. The doctor-patient relationship, even indirect, is fiduciary and must take precedence over economic or personal influences. 4D. The dental consultant must regard 'standard of care' the same for all providers" [2].

To not provide coverage for these procedures would be a disservice to my patient and your client. To not allow benefits could be taken as Bad Faith Coverage. According to the standard of care in dentistry, reasonable care and diligence includes patient examination. To diagnose a patient's or client's dental needs without an examination is below the standard of care per se [5].

Failure to allow benefits or needed treatment would be taken as Bad Faith Insurance and would have to be reported to the _____ State Department of Insurance.

Again, I understand that at times it is hard to determine benefits without seeing the patient. However, to not provide coverage for these procedures would be a disservice to my patient and your client.

Thank you for your immediate attention and cooperation in providing proper care for your client and my patient, _____.

Sincerely,

Nonpayment After Reliance on Estimation of Benefits

There are also occasions where the insurance company will state in their EOB that they will pay for a procedure and then deny payment upon receipt of the dental claim.

It is always surprising at the insurance company's boldness to refuse payment after they have issued an EOB that you and the patient have relied on to proceed with the treatment decided upon. This could be with an insurance company that you are or are not in contract with to accept their terms of payment.

To Whom It May Concern:

Per your letter of _____, I am surprised that you have denied benefits after pre-authorizing for the treatment rendered. (*If not contracted with insurance company*) It must be pointed out that the _____ Insurance has not been contracted with myself or this office. Therefore, we are not held to any proposed negotiated rate that ___(Ins. Co.)_____ may have with other providers.)

It must also be pointed out that you have pre-authorized this treatment (see enclosed copy) upon which I, my office, and your client, _____ have detrimentally relied upon. To now disallow benefits is clearly seen as a fraudulent misrepresentation of your willingness to abide by your own representations and admissions. This is also a clear case of Bad Faith Insurance of which I must inform my patient and your client, _____. This may necessitate a report to the _____ State Department of Insurance.

Also, you should be aware that dental consultants should abide by the American Association of Dental Consultants Code of Ethics. As stated in Principle 4, "4B. The ethical aspects of dental consultant duties must always take precedence over economic aspects. 4C. The doctor-patient relationship, even indirect, is fiduciary and must take precedence over economic or personal influences" [2].

Thank you for your immediate attention in providing proper previously approved benefits for my patient and your client, _____.

Sincerely,

Insurance Fee Schedule for Non-covered Services

Even though many states have enacted laws to various degrees that prevent insurance companies from forcing dentists to accept the insurance fee schedule for procedures that are not covered or are beyond the patients benefit level, insurance companies still attempt to enforce their fee schedules in such situations. This is very state specific. Some states have enacted very strong legislature "cap laws" to prevent such insurance company practices, while others like New York have very weak legislature regulating the dental insurance company. There is also the distinction of whether the patient's insurance is self-funded or not. Per your jurisdiction, self-funded employee benefit plans may not be included in such "cap laws" since they may not be considered an insurance company. Many times, per the provider contact you signed, the insurance company may have a clause that you provide 20–30% discount or must abide by the contracted fee schedule for procedures not covered by the insurance company. This type of clause relates to that treatment that is beyond the maximum yearly limit benefit or is not on the agreed-to fee schedule. This is an attempt by the insurance company to circumvent state "cap laws." If you believe you are entitled to your UCR fee on a non-covered service, the letter below needs to be adapted to your state's laws on this issue.

To Whom It May Concern:
Upon review of my contract, there is no mention of having to charge _____ (insurance company) fees for services that _____ (insurance co.) is not covering. It does say a 30% discount of the UCR fee for services not on the insurance fee schedule.

In accordance with Section 4224(d)(1) and/or Section 2324 of the New York State Insurance Law, requiring discounts for non-covered services is a direct violation as defined under Section 2402(b) of the Insurance Law [6, 7]. (Your state most likely have similar laws.)

Hence, it is within the _____ State Insurance Law that a provider may charge his or her UCR fee for services and/or devices not covered by insurance.

Thank you for your continued efforts to provide proper dental care benefits for my patient and your client _____.

Sincerely,

Request of Refund from an Insurance Company You Do Not Participate

Insurance companies perform a yearly audit of their accounts payable. You may receive a letter that informs you that you have been mistakenly paid or overpaid without your misrepresentation of treatment and billing and without your knowledge of the mistake. The insurance company due to their unilateral mistake is not entitled to a refund. However, most provider contracts allow for audits and requests of money. In such situations and if not repaid, the amount sought by the insurance company that was overpaid or paid by mistake will be withheld from future payments from that insurance company. If you are not a contracted provider with the insurance company, you most likely would not have to pay the requested refund depending on the situation.

Dear _____,

I am writing in response to your letter requesting that I return monies paid on behalf of a client of _____. I am writing to request that you cease and desist from contacting me regarding monies the company dental plan may be owed by the company's client. I further request that you terminate immediately any collection actions initiated against me. I am not the company's debtor, but am a creditor against whom no action can lie.

It is inappropriate for you to contact any dentist regarding matters that solely involves the company and its client. In situations in which the dentist is not a contractor (PPO provider) with the company, or any affiliated benefit-related company, any such request for reimbursement properly should be addressed directly to the company's client. As I am not under any contract with the company's dental plan, what the company plan is entitled to or to be determined by the company's policy contract with its client, and _____ State Law. Regardless, it does not involve me. Only the company's client can dispute or confirm that monies were improperly paid, and any refund would be due solely from the client and not from his or her dentist.

It is widely held that an insurance carrier is not entitled to recover an overpayment made to an incorrect third-party creditor when 1) that payment was made solely due to the insurer's mistake, 2) the mistake was not induced by a misrepresentation of the third-party creditor, and 3) the third-party creditor acted in good faith without prior knowledge of the mistake. See, e.g. St. Mary's Med. Ctr. V. United Farm Bureau, 624 N.E.2d 939 (Ind. App. 1 Dist. 1993); time Ins. V. Fulton-DeKalb Hosp. Auth., 211 Ga. App. 4, 438 E.2d 149 (Ga. App.1993); Lincoln Nat. Live v. Brown Schools, 757 S. W. 2d 493 (Neb.Sup. Ct. 1971); Mutual Benefit Life Insurance co. v. Lindenman, 911 F. Supp. 619 (EDNY, 1995); New York Life Ins. Co. v. Guttenplan, 30 N.Y.S. 2d 430; and Prudential Ins. Co. of America v. Couch, 376 S.E.2d 104 (W. Va. Sup. Ct. of App. 1988).

I trust that I will not hear from you again regarding this matter.

Sincerely,

When the Insurance Company Fails to Pay

There are times when the insurance company fails to pay. The insurance coordinator in your office has called and told they never received the claim, need more information, or are behind in sending payments. The first two reasons for delays are easy to fix by resending the claim with any additional requested information. The last is a little more involved. Many states (check your jurisdiction) have a limit on how long an insurance company can delay payment. New York Prompt Payment Law (Insurance Law Section 3224-a) states that the insurance company has 45 days to deny a claim and 45 days to pay an undisputed claim [8].

To Whom It May Concern:

I submitted a claim for _____ on __(Date)__. As of the above date payment has not been received. Please beware of ___(State Law)__, which states that payment or denial must be made within __(number of days your jurisdiction allows)__.

Payment must be received within __(number of days)__ of the above date or I must advise my patient, your client, to notify the _____ State Insurance Department for Bad Faith Coverage and failure to comply with _____ State Law.

Thank you for your immediate cooperation.

Sincerely,

References

1 American Dental Association Current Dental Terminology Code Book (CDT 2017: Dental Procedure Codes), pp. 22, 24.
2 American Association of Dental Consultants, Code of Ethics, 2017. https://www.aadc.org/aboutus/codeofethics (accessed 10 June 2018).
3 American Dental Association Current Dental Terminology Code Book (CDT 2017: Dental Procedure Codes), p. 15.
4 American Dental Association Current Dental Terminology Code Book (CDT 2017: Dental Procedure Codes), p. 39.

5 Graskemper, J.P. (2004). Standard of care in dentistry: where did it come from? How has it evolved? *Journal of the American Dental Association* 135: 1449.

6 New York State Law, Office of General Counsel, Department of Financial Services N.Y. Ins. Law §§ 2324 & 4224; Inducement to Purchase Insurance, 15 October 2004. https://www.dfs.ny.gov/insurance/ogco2004/rg041014.htm (accessed 10 June 2018).

7 New York State Law, Office of General Counsel, Department of Financial Services Rebating, Insurance Law Section 2324, 28 February 2000. https://www.dfs.ny.gov/insurance/ogco2000/rg000211.htm (accessed 10 June 2018).

8 New York State Law, Office of General Counsel, Department of Financial Services, New York Insurance Law § 3224-a, 5 May 2011. https://www.dfs.ny.gov/insurance/ogco2011/rg110503.htm (accessed 10 June 2018).

6

Leadership to Interface with Your Community

Nothing great was ever achieved without enthusiasm.
Ralph Waldo Emerson

It's never too late to be what you might have been.
George Eliot

The interface of you and your practice with your community is one of the best practice builders to ensure long-term practice growth. Leading a practice to be the best it can be within the community has two prongs of effort: internal and external. Internally is the office space, equipment, and office street appeal. Externally is the marketing, advertising, social media, and community involvement.

Internally is most important because even with over-the-top external marketing, if the practice does not appear to be what is expected based on that marketing, the patient will become disheartened and question their choice of dentist. Always keep the office very clean and fresh looking. All employees should be presentable, courteous, helpful, and above all knowledgeable. It can be simply the way a staff member answers the phone that could be a turn off to a new patient.

True Case (11)
Many times, when calling an office to hear the greeting of "Doctor's office" leaves a lot to be desired to make a patient feel welcome even if it is a longtime patient. The new or existing patient may question if they called the right doctor's office. Would it not be better to answer the phone: "Good Morning, Dr. Smith's office or South Country Dental Group. This is Susan. How may I help you?"

Leadership and Communication in Dentistry, First Edition. Joseph P. Graskemper.
© 2019 John Wiley & Sons, Inc. Published 2019 by John Wiley & Sons, Inc.

I highly recommend several things to help maintain the office looking fresh and clean:

1) Have the windows washed on a regular basis, preferably monthly inside and out.
2) Maintain the magazine materials to be up to date and in good shape. No torn, crumpled, or folded pages.
3) Have the walls touched up on a yearly basis and repainted even if in the same color every 5–10 years, depending on wear.
4) Even if you have a cleaning service to do floors and bathrooms, make sure they are maintained or replaced when needed.
5) Make sure all seating areas including office, waiting room, and operatory chairs are in good repair and presentable.
6) The outside of the building or office space you are occupying is well maintained.
7) Make sure all equipment is clean and in good working order.

Many dentists buy the latest equipment and use it diligently. Over time the equipment will begin to look well used and dated. Patients notice the smallest of things when it comes to their impression of whether they have chosen the right dentist. All equipment should be properly maintained and kept clean. Patients notice if computer equipment and software is up to date and operating properly.

Patients notice if you take leadership in maintaining the office. You as the owner/dentist/leader are responsible for taking the lead in making sure the inside and the outside of your practice is the image you want patients to remember you by.

Externally, there many articles, books, blogs, and practice management consultants all trying to guide and help dentists promote their practices through their marketing, advertising, social media, and websites. When initiating a relationship with a marketing company, be very sure that your culture/brand remains intact and you maintain an ethical, professional image. Branding begins with how you perceive your self and your practice and how you project that within your community. Branding extends to how you live and the way you communicate and interact with others. Even the way you spend money within your practice's community says a lot about you. Since most small practices are an extension of the owner(s), the images within the community of what you do and how you act brand you and your practice. If you dress shabbily, prospective new patients in the community will think you provide shabby dentistry. You are the brand!

Many of the newer marketing promotions tend to give dentistry a merchant's image of professional services. Marketing of a successful practice was covered in part in my first book, *Professional Responsibility in Dentistry: A Practical Guide to Law and Ethics*. Since its publication, social media has had extreme growth.

In 2012, it was found that just 22% said they had used online reviews once or more. In 2014, however, this percentage jumped to 42% – marking a 68% increase from 2013. Another very interesting survey result was the statistic that points to the growing importance of review sites. It found that nearly half of respondents (44%) said they would consider going to an out-of-network doctor if their reviews were better than those of in-network doctors. This is a significant change from 2013 when just 26% of respondents said they'd be willing to go out-of-network because of more favorable reviews. The shift in patient sentiment here seems to reflect a growing reliance on online physician reviews over other factors when selecting a healthcare provider [1].

Therefore, you must routinely review various review sites such as Yelp, Marketcircle, Healthgrades, etc. I highly recommend you Google yourself to check on reviews. Many of the review sites offer a service, usually at no charge, to alert you when a review has been made on their service. A complete discussion of social media is the beyond the scope of this book. You must protect your "webutation."

There are also online consultations services available for dentists to sign up as an online dental advisor to answer questions from individuals seeking dental information. If you decide to foray into the online consultations, beware that whenever a dentist gives an individual a dental opinion upon which the individual may reasonably relies on, a cyber doctor–patient relationship may have formed. This could leave the dentist open to malpractice allegations.

Search engine optimization (SEO) has become very popular to promote the dental practice. Be very careful to question the methods your selected SEO use to promote your practice online. The SEO that you have subscribed to may be applying merchant-type tactics and processes that may not seem professional.

Everyone likes a good review, but what to do about a bad review can be troubling. If handled the wrong way, it will only make the situation worse. Never discuss a patient's dental care online because Health Insurance Portability and Accountability Act (HIPAA) and doctor–patient confidentiality laws. The more you put online defending or answering the negative review, the higher up the list it goes, making it one of the first things people see when searching for you or your practice. Wait 24 hours to let the patient and your self to calm down and allow you to leave emotions out of the discussion. Try to reach out to the patient and contact them in a very calm manner and see if you can resolve their problem with the hope that they take down the post. The main thing is to remain calm, even if it means remaking or retreating the patient at no further charge. You can post general information regarding patient care or a dental procedure in general terms without reference to the patient, or seek more positive posts, such that you dilute the negative. As the saying goes, "The solution to pollution is dilution." If you are asking for a review from a patient, be very sure you will receive the review you were anticipating.

True Case (12)

For a dentist wanting to have more online reviews, he and the staff requested patient reviews. One patient, having had endodontic therapy and a crown, had soreness a couple of months later. The dentist checked the tooth and all appeared OK. The patient then went home and posted a negative review.

Therefore, be very careful when getting involved in social media regarding your office or yourself. It is hard to unfriend or block a patient after they have gotten too intrusive, abrasive, or personal.

What you post on a site is just as important as how you post the information. Always keep your practice culture/brand at the forefront. The images you post are only viewed for a few seconds but may have a lasting memory. Do not post politics, religion, or invasive procedures that show a little too much. Beware of staff and patient privacy issues while following all HIPAA regulations, and do not use stolen or borrowed content including pictures of public figures, celebrities, and other advertisements or photos.

Posting information should be about the practice, your staff (with the person's consent), and yourself showing the personality/culture/branding of the office and not just about the doctor. With permission, share staff and doctor information regarding charities in which they are involved, wishing staff members happy birthday. Hobbies, volunteerism, and sports show the human side of the team. There are many positive things that can be shared to make a connection to those you are reaching out to.

A good guideline (THINK) to be considered before posting any information:

Is it True?
Is it Helpful?
It is Inspiring?
Is it Necessary?
Is it Kind?

Therefore, THINK about the impression your posted information will make on others by viewing your post from the perspective of a new patient.

There are many other ways to communicate and take leadership in the community. Joining a community service organization that you believe in immediately connects you to many people in the community with like interests. Do not join only to get patients since that could easily be taken that you have false intentions and only joined to be self-serving. If you are not truly engaged in the efforts of the chosen community service, it could possibly hurt you and your practice more than help it. There are many great service organizations such as Kiwanis, Rotary, Lions, or Elks and various other organizations that help the local community like the Chamber of Commerce.

Being part of the community around your office is very important. It can be done easily by using the various merchants, grocery stores, and restaurants in the area and become familiar with the other small business owners. Give dental hygiene kits with your name on it to the local pharmacies, hotels, and real estate offices to be given to their customers if in need. Whenever there is a fundraiser by a local church, synagogue, temple, school, or athletic club, be sure to pitch in with an ad for their program or journal. Placing a small ad for the various fundraisers keeps your practice in front of those in the community who are possible new patients. There are also many golf outing fundraisers that request an ad or tee sign. These are usually inexpensive and are another way to show community support. It also allows you to show those who are patients that you support the community that supports you. These are all very important communications to show your community that you are a leader within the community – a community that supports you and your practice.

True Case (13)
A dentist who invested time and money in local fundraisers got to know many fellow members of the community. One of the fellow volunteers at several of the fundraisers got to know the dentist through his support of the various organizations. Although she was not a patient of the dentist at the time, she referred many people to his office who all became patients. She later became a patient and continues to refer many people to the dentist's office.

Every professional should be aware that having a professional degree, more times than not, is held more accountable, admired, and respected due to having the initials "Dr." in front of their name. Due to your higher professional education, many in the community will default to you as a leader within the community. You must connect with the community as a leader.

Reference

1 Leslie, J. Patient use of online reviews – 2014. https://www.softwareadvice.com/resources/medical-online-reviews-report-2014 (accessed 16 June 2012).

Section 2

Leadership, Communication, and Success for Your Practice

To have a successful dental practice the dentist must have the capability to lead both the patients and the staff. Therefore this section is separated into two parts that give insight to the dentist who wants to lead patients using proper communications tools to make the practice the best it can be.

Leadership and Communication in Dentistry, First Edition. Joseph P. Graskemper.
© 2019 John Wiley & Sons, Inc. Published 2019 by John Wiley & Sons, Inc.

Part I: Your Patients

7

Listening

> *Earn your leadership every day.*
> **Michael Jordan**

> *Great minds discuss ideas,*
> *average minds discuss events,*
> *small minds discuss people.*
> **Eleanor Roosevelt**

Your patients are the lifeblood of your practice. And new patients are the heart of it. Leading your staff to become fully engaged in having new patients choose your office should be constantly at the forefront of all the staff. Just like large fast food chains or any other successful business based on taking orders or making an appointment, it must be made as easy as possible. If your phone lines are always full, you may think that is a good thing. But are the phone lines always busy because staff is making personal calls, long "on-hold" sessions with an insurance company, or existing patient insurance inquiries? When the lines are full, new patients cannot get through. A new patient emergency will simply call another office to make that emergency appointment.

So, the first thing to properly lead your patient is to have the opportunity to do so – easily get them their first appointment. Make sure you have enough lines available. Most phone services can give a report on how many times your lines are full. You must also have the entire staff trained on how to answer the phone. It is not just a front office job duty, but the whole office must be involved when the phone rings. Any phone call should not be allowed to ring more than three times. You as the leader of the office must be part of this endeavor and lead the staff on the importance of making that first appointment. Also make sure your website/social media has appointment-making capability. If website/social media is being used, follow all legal Health Insurance Portability and Accountability Act (HIPAA) and privacy laws and regulations.

Leadership and Communication in Dentistry, First Edition. Joseph P. Graskemper.
© 2019 John Wiley & Sons, Inc. Published 2019 by John Wiley & Sons, Inc.

Once the new patient enters your office and is seated, you need to use leadership skills to properly communicate your competence in providing the proper care of the patient's concerns. Your competence level will lead the patient to place trust in you as their dental healthcare provider. Many times that level of trust has been preconceived by the patient due to your marketing or how that patient chose your office. Hence, it is very important to make sure any marketing of you or your practice promotes the image you want patients to have. If your marketing is merchant-like and not on the level of professionalism, the new patient will have a consumer-based rather than a patient-based image of the service and care they will receive. In other words, they will be buying a dental procedure rather than seeking dental care from a professional who they trust will have their best interests in the forefront of their care.

The presentation of you and your office must be a statement of professionalism. The décor of your office and the presentation of your staff and yourself all make an image to the patient of you and what your practice is all about. It communicates indirectly to the patient regarding the care they are about to receive.

True Case (14)

A parent took their child to the dentist office. While waiting to get attention from the receptionist in order to fill out the office forms, he noticed that the staff was too busy telling stories about the recent weekend for a couple of minutes before acknowledging him. He became a little concerned. Once the forms were done, he and his child were led to an operatory. The floor was well worn and the dental chair had a small hole in it. It appeared clean but could be questioned. He became a little more concerned. The dentist enters the operatory wearing well-worn shoes, wrinkled pants, and wrinkled short sleeve scrub top. When the dentist introduced himself, his breath smelt like burnt coffee. The dentist then said the assistant will take an X-ray. He then returned and told the patient and the parent that the tooth needs to come out. The parent decided to make an appointment with no intention of ever returning to that office. As you can see a lot was communicated to the parent and child without the dentist saying much.

Being a new dentist, your first encounter with the patient should be a greeting or a welcome to the practice and a concern regarding the reason they came to see you. When entering the operatory, you should have a smile and offer a handshake or a slight touching of the shoulder to make connection with the patient. This is very important to show the patient that you are happy to see them, no matter what the problem may be. Using the body language of a handshake or touching on the shoulder signals that you are there with them and for them. With these signs of welcome and acceptance of the patient, listening may now begin. As the saying goes, "God gave you 2 ears and 1 mouth so you can listen twice as much as you talk." Your full attention must be given to the patient, so you are not just hearing them but truly listening to their wants, needs, desires, fears, concerns, questions, and misunderstandings. This will allow you to address their needs and wants better and clarify any misunderstandings of their needs based on misconceptions. As the leader of their dental care, you lead the patient by relieving the patient's anxiety, apprehension, and cautions. Proper listening allows you to lead the patient to proper treatment plan decisions and reassurance that you and your office will stay focused on his or her well-being.

True Case (15)

An elderly patient presented with severe periodontal disease that has resulted in all teeth being non-restorable. The patient's teeth would actually move and cause considerable pain upon biting. The patient understood the need for immediate dentures, and the dentist, after a thorough discussion of what the patient should expect with a valid consent, began treatment. Once all the teeth were extracted and the immediate dentures placed, the patient over the next few months complained about how the dentures were getting loose. Again, the dentist explained the resorption and provided soft temporary relines for her comfort as needed. At one of these appointments, the patient asked if he could refer her "to someone who knew what they are doing." The dentist, although very frustrated with the patient, was courteous and friendly while maintaining many soft relines, till six months have passed. Upon placing the final reline, the patient stated: "We make a good team, don't we doc?"

Your full attention is needed to fully understand the patient and the reason they are there. It is normal to try and think of the answers to their problems before they have completed their side of the story, which can sometimes be quite lengthy. But being quiet and listening to the end allows the patient to build trust in you before you even speak. This is due to the patient subconsciously reading your body language. The influence of body language is beyond the scope of this book, so I advise you to pick up one of the many books on the subject. You will quickly learn that your nonverbal communication, including but not limited to, facial expressions, eye movement, hand gestures, and body posture convey a lot of information to the patient even before you say your first word. Albert Mehrabian in 1971 researched the amount being communicated nonverbally. He found that 55% of communication is derived through nonverbal communication as in body language, 38% is the tone of voice, and only 7% is the actual words spoken [1]. Believing nonverbal communication more than verbal communication makes the nonverbal communication very important to motivate a patient to seek proper dental care [2].

Hence, a lot of communication is made without talking. Sometimes, just keeping a professional, friendly demeanor and treating the patient with kindness goes a lot further than you may think.

True Case (16)

A young dentist bought out an older dentist's practice. The older dentist wore a scrub top and casual pants and causal shoes. The young dentist continued that image for a couple of years. He then decided to move it up a notch. He redecorated the office, had the staff in color coordinated scrubs, and started wearing a tie, dress shirt with dress pants, dress shoes, and a white clinic coat. After two months with new images of authority and confidence, his case acceptance went up over 30%. This new image communicated professionalism and care – care about how the office looked, the way he looked, and the way his staff looked. The patients felt they could trust him because it all showed he cared.

Once the patient has been seated and begins to tell their story, the dentist and the staff must be good listeners. Preparing for the patient interaction, the SMILES approach can be used:

Smile – Smiling is the universal sign of friendliness. Ninety-three percent of anxious patient (which are most patients to some degree) prefer a provider to be friendly [3]. Smiling often and sincerely when greeting the patient either for the first time or on every appointment builds a trusting doctor–patient relationship.

Make contact – Making contact with the patient reassures the patient of a caring attitude. Any contact with the patient should be limited to a handshake or a soft touch on the shoulder to reassure the patient. The handshake should be firm but not crushing and appropriate to the patient's size and sex. Touching should never happen on the torso, arms, or legs.

Incline toward the patient – Leaning slightly toward the patient to show interest in what they are saying. It is a sign of your attentiveness to their needs to explain their situation.

Lower hands – Keeping your hands lowered or in your lap prevents you from making unwanted gestures or movements. Open arms are much more welcoming than crossed arms.

Eye contact – Perhaps it is one of the most important nonverbal communications that occurs. It is the most universal sign of trust and integrity in a doctor–patient relationship. It is not to be a stare-down with the patient but taking a pause in data collection and entry and making eye contact helps build trust. Also, to help keep your attention, look in one rather than both of the patient's eyes to help you focus on the patient's words, connotations, and body language.

Sit – Sitting down with the patient will relieve any patient feeling of an intimidating or overbearing provider. It also means you have taken the time to sit and listen as compared with standing with your feet angled toward the door as if you are ready to leave as soon as you have arrived [4].

Now that you have set the stage for a successful patient encounter, you can focus on the patient with your full attention.

There are many barriers to effective listening: time, effort, message overload, rapid thought, psychological noise, physical noise, hearing problems, faulty assumptions, emphasis on talk, and cultural differences [5].

Time being a big factor in the dental office, you have specific time limitations to listen, discuss, and treat the patient, especially in a very busy practice with tight scheduling and of course the need to produce. However, taking the time now with the patient to allow the patient to build trust in you allows you to better understand the patient on many levels. It takes time to build a trusting doctor–patient relationship by which you can lead the patient to understanding and accepting your proposed dental care. It also will save time later in the treatment sessions because the patient has full trust in you. The time and effort spent at the treatment discussion phase will be well spent because you took the time to understand the patient's wants and educated them about their needs. This allows for patient needs to become patient wants.

Message overload occurs when too many outside messages interrupt your listening endeavor. Parts of the patient's message will be lost due to staff and phone call interruptions. The staff must understand that your time with the patient should not be interrupted unless there is an eminent and immediate need. The whole dental team must work together to focus on the patient's concerns and understanding of their dental problem or situation.

Rapid thoughts occur when the dentist is already evaluating the patient's problems without fully listening to the patient, interrupting them with immediate solutions, or anticipating what the patient will say next by interjecting the patient's next word. Because the dentist is able to understand the problem faster and easier than the patient is able to describe or explain it, it is easier for the dentist to move much faster to the solution than the patient. He or she will be tempted to interrupt the patient to show how much they know to quickly treat the patient. It is better to allow the patient to fully explain their concerns. With today's time constraints, if it is taking more time than you can allow to remain on schedule, and you believe you understand the concern or problem, simply say, "You're way ahead of me. May I take a look to catch up to you?" There is also the interference of psychological and physical noise that must be dealt with if trust is to develop between doctor and patient.

Psychological noise is all the thoughts that interfere with you fully listening to the patient. We all have thoughts roaming around in the back of our minds while talking or listening. When those thoughts overtake the immediate need to listen, you are merely hearing the patient and not truly listening. As a leader you must master the art of placing this interfering psychological noise into a quiet mode while you direct your attention to the patient in front of you. This is also very important when talking to your staff as a group or as individuals. A very easy way to accomplish that is to maintain eye-to-eye contact. As mentioned before, keeping eye contact while listening will help you focus on what the patient is saying. This lets the patient know you are listening and focused on their concerns.

Physical noise is everywhere in the dental office: ringing phones, the background music, and overhearing how the staff is speaking to each other and to patients in another operatory. Overhearing the staff also adds to psychological noise since it draws your thought processes to that conversation. As a leader you need to trust in yourself that you have trained your staff to properly handle that outside interference and keeping it at a minimum.

Hearing problems are an obvious barrier to proper listening. It is well known that dentists may have slight hearing loss due to long-term exposure to high-speed handpiece noise [6]. So, if you missed what the patient said or if you lost focus, ask a question to clarify your understanding and to verify your listening. Patients also have hearing problems, some of whom will not admit to their faulty hearing. If you notice you are losing connection with the patients' hearing, again ask a question if they understood what you just said to verify communication.

Faulty assumptions occur almost all the time due to the listener's biases. This may be based on the stereotyping of a patient's appearance, behavior, or speech. It may also occur with a patient with a reoccurring problem that the dentist precon-cludes the needed treatment before fully listening to the patient. During the diagnosis of a problem, dentist sometimes jump ahead of the patient's full story based on the dentist's experience thinking he or she understands the patient's problem before the patient is even finished telling the dentist what the patient's problem is. This may lead to a faulty diagnosis and subsequent unneeded treatment.

Emphasis on what one is saying is a normal occurrence in most conversations. Both sides want to be heard and control the direction of the conversation. Allow the patient to talk and emphasize their concern or problem so that you may fully understand the patient and lead them. They will not follow your treatment suggestions or listen to you unless they believe you fully understand their need. This emphasis is more important than you speaking too soon so as to cut the patient short. Patients will take that as you not being truly concerned or caring.

Cultural differences are evident with many different languages that may be hard to understand. Also, various cultures place different importance on dental care. To lead a culturally different patient, you must first understand their dental understanding that I call the "Dental IQ" [7]. Once you understand where the patient's "Dental IQ" is then, you can begin to lead them to a higher level to properly treat them. It is normal for a patient to filter the communication through their personal perspective [8]. You must understand the patient's mindset regarding dental care. With a clear understanding of the patient, you can then lead them to proper treatment planning decision making.

True Case (17)
A mother brought her 21-year-old daughter to see the dentist due to pain. The mother (before the HIPAA), explained to the dentist that everyone in the family usually gets their dentures by the time they are 25. Her daughter being 21, it was now her daughter's time to get dentures. Additionally, the cost of ideal dental treatment was well beyond the family's financial abilities. The daughter, having several missing teeth and several that were severely carious, agreed with the mother. The dentist discussed the importance of trying to keep a few teeth for retention of a partial denture and/or reduce the amount of ridge resorption that will take place over time if a denture were made. The dentist relieved the pain and had the daughter and mother back to discuss some options to save some teeth, at a cost no more than that of a denture. A provisional partial denture was made. By taking the time to listen and communicate with the patient, and mother in this case, the dentist was able to raise the patient's dental understanding ("Dental IQ") and provide a great service for the daughter [9].

Bridging the cultural divide can be achieved by being attentive to the following strategies [8]:

Develop mindfulness – Be consciously aware of cultural differences and be aware that the assumptions of both patient and doctor may be and probably are different. The loss of a tooth is viewed very differently around the world.

Be flexible – You may have to adapt and change to accommodate the perceptions and assumptions of the patient to allow the patient to fulfill their dental needs. Patients will allow you to lead when you match the patient's idea of what a good dentist leader should be. It may not be what is ideal treatment under your standards, but if you get the patient to just move a little closer to understanding their dental needs, raising their "Dental IQ," you have helped that patient.

Tolerate uncertainty and ambiguity – Take the time and be patient. Some patients may need to think about it or even need a second consultation appointment to understand and become motivated. It takes time to break down barriers of long standing.

Resist stereotyping and making negative judgments about others – Do not become defensive in your discussion with the patient. Rather you should be open, confirmatory, and supportive in discussing the patient's needs. This allows you to gently lead the patient to good decision making rather than being argumentative and overbearing. Never prejudge a patient's wants, understandings, or financial abilities by giving a lesser treatment plan. You can always adapt and adjust the treatment plan to the patient's understanding and financial abilities.

Ask questions – You must ask questions to understand the patient's beliefs regarding their oral health. Try to understand the reasoning of their opinion by seeking additional information and meaning as to why they have such an opinion. If you do not ask, you will never know and hence never lead them to the proper decision. Sharing is caring!

Be other oriented – Be sensitive, understanding, and emphatic of the patient and not to marginalize an uninformed opinion. Put yourself in their shoes to understand where the patient is coming from. Through understanding of the patient's viewpoint, you can then educate and elevate the patient "Dental IQ."

To improve your listening ability for patients and staff, here are nine pointers to become a better listener:

1) There is a lot to listen for in a conversation. Listen for the patient's wants, needs, desires, fears, concerns, questions, and misunderstandings. The more you understand the patient, the better you may properly respond.

2) Better to listen with an understanding of all the facets of the conversation, such as any underlying tension, frustration, or embarrassment.

3) Shut off the psychological noise and focus on the patient.

4) Most people repeat what is important to them so the listener is sure to get it. Many people often repeat a message they are trying to relay three times: once to get your attention, once to see if you are hearing it, and a third time to make sure you were listening. The message may be repeated three times in different ways or formats. Listen for the repeat!

5) Listen for what is not being said or contains false understandings or beliefs.

6) Listen for why the patient is there. Why did they come to the office? What was their motivation to seek dental care at that moment?

7) A good listener will not respond quickly or finish the patient's sentences. Let a little silence, only moments to let the mind gather a proper response. Not every statement by the patient needs to be responded to. Let the patient to get it all out. They will be more comfortable and will be more likely to trust your response.

8) A good listener asks good questions because they took the time to truly understand what the patient was saying. Not just statements made to the patient but questions also may be enlightening to the patient and uncover a better understanding.

9) While listening, take inventory of your own physical reactions. Everyone has some biases, prejudgments, prejudices, thoughts, and motives. To be a great listener and leader, these immediate thoughts must be eliminated to allow the listener to embrace what is being said. It is only after the patient

has fully disclosed their situation and you have fully listened that these thoughts may have a basis. To allow those thoughts to enter into the act of listening affects the reception of what is being said [10].

Responding is just as important as listening. During the conversation, there should be small verbal and nonverbal cues that signal attention and encourage the patient to continue talking. Some verbal cues are: "Yeah," Uh-huh," Oh, really?," "I see." Some nonverbal cues are eye contact, head nods, smiles, and eyebrow raising [11].

Listening is only part of the equation to lead your patient.

There are many facets that must be taken into account in leading the patient to a proper understanding and wanting to have the necessary treatment. You must not only listen with the patient but also educate and then motivate the patient.

To educate the patient takes more than just telling the patient what needs to be done. You need to educate the patient by involving them in the treatment plan discussion. It is the incorporation of the patient into the diagnosing phase that educates the patient, whereby the patient will build trust in your leadership to the desired treatment plan. This is called co-diagnosis: the involvement of the patient through education to understand not just the need for treatment but also why the treatment is needed. By involving the patient to this level, the patient will then be more motivated, and hence their "Dental IQ" or awareness is raised, allowing the patient to better understand and appreciate the needed care, creating a dental want rather than just fulfilling a dental need [12]. There are many software programs, dental models, and enlarged images of radiographs and intraoral photographs that are available to lead the treatment discussion.

Each visit should begin with information about what is going to be done and what the patient should expect. This is a continuous education of the patient such that by the second or third appointment, depending on their "Dental IQ," the patient will fully understand what is being done and fully knowledgeable of what to expect. This also builds trust in the doctor–patient relationship. So, at the beginning of an appointment, you should state what is being done in very simple terms.

True Case (Example) (18)

After the greeting, "We're doing a crown and 2 fillings on the lower right side. First, I am going to place some pre-numbing salve on the area and then get that area numb. You will feel a little pinch and then some pressure and I will shake the area as I do it. Half of your tongue and lower jaw will be asleep and may feel a little funny to swallow. The crown is on a back tooth and the other 2 fillings are on the side teeth. If you need me to stop or having a problem, simply raise your hand and I will stop. Do you have any questions?" This opens the door for the patient to discuss any hesitancies or questions they may have.

Not every person learns the same way. Some are receptive to visual images such as patient education programs showing dental images and videos, while others only need an explanation in common terms to understand the proposed treatment. Patient education programs, of which there are many, are easy and very descriptive. Explaining necessary treatment in common terms takes a little more effort. Patients do not understand mesial and distal. They understand front and back. Just telling a patient they need a root canal does not do much for the patient other than to make them cringe. Better to show them via the enlarged radiographic image or the patient education program and explain the benefits of the procedure in common terms.

True Case (19)

A patient comes to the office for the first time due to pain on the lower right side. After a review of the medical/dental history, it is discovered that the patient has not been to a dentist for eight years. It is very important to find out why: phobia, financial, or just scared from prior experiences or being away from dental care for a long time worrying about how bad it is. This takes time and in doing so builds the patient's trust in you. You find it is due to fear of pain. But now the pain is so bad that they are forced to seek care. Before even taking a radiograph, this patient's concern must be listened to and understood before going any further. Discussion must be had to relieve the patient's fear and allow you to lead the patient forward to the proposed treatment, a root canal. With this understanding, a simple explanation of a root canal is the numbing of the area and removing the nerve of the tooth like a wick out of a candle and then filling in the area with a special material.

It is very important to take the time during your first contact with the patient to fully engage the patient in the discussion. Sometimes it is better to discuss the outcome first rather than the treatment itself. I call this "backward diagnosing." In other words, discuss the patient's dental concerns not from the point of how you will do it but from the viewpoint of the patient – what will it be like when we're done. In the above example discuss the relief of pain and the saving of the tooth before discussing the manner in which it is done. This "backward diagnosing" works well on patients who have in the past centered their thoughts on the doing of the procedure and not on the benefits of the procedure. Giving the patient the aftertreatment value before discussing the need for the procedure allows the patient to focus on the benefits of treatment rather than the procedure itself. Once this change in viewpoint is accomplished, the patient will become more active in their dental care and actually become motivated.

The motivation of a patient is based on four pillars: an attainable goal, an understanding of the goal to attain it, a change in attitude to obtain the goal, and the patient's personal perceived value in reaching the goal (see Chapter 8).

Be aware that the outcomes of the patient and doctor may be different. The dentist's outcome may be more technical and the patient's may be more health or cosmetic related. In your discussion, be sure to match your skills and communication to the patient and their needs technically, emotionally, and financially. Be careful *not* to match the patient needs to your skills. You may be very good at veneers. But does every patient need veneers to have that perfect smile as you perceive it, and not what the patient perceives as to what they want their smile to be?

True Case (20)

A patient came in for a second opinion to close a small 1 mm diastema between teeth #8 and #9. All of the other teeth have no restorations and in perfect alignment. She has already been to two other dental offices with the recommendation of porcelain veneers for teeth #6 through #11 "to make it all uniform." Upon examination, it was suggested that some cosmetic bonding be placed on both teeth to close the space. The patient agreed to "give it a try." The patient ended up very happy and became one of the largest referral sources in the practice.

The patient must be given a goal or end point of treatment in order for there to be any improvement for the patient. The goal may be anything from straighter teeth or more beautiful smile or be able to eat better or without pain. These are goals that most people want. These wants come with some basic dental needs (extractions, root canal therapy, restorations) that must be done to achieve the patient's wants. But how do we turn those needs into wants? Proper communication can lead the patient to the intended goal. Remember no one really needs dentistry other than relief of pain, so most dental expenditures are discretionary. That means dental dollars are competing with vacation dollars, new car dollars, new electronics dollars, etc. First and foremost, the patient must understand the immediate and long-term benefits of treatment and the risks of no treatment. The value of the proposed treatment plan must be presented to give the goal its intended importance. The patient should feel somewhat inspired, which is the feeling of value the patient feels while working toward the patient-centered, patient-decided goal. Value is judged by the service or the product received. To have a patient motivated, the value must be greater than or equal to the service received. He or she must believe they are receiving more than their money's worth.

For some people, it may have to be presented as the fear of losing something to motivate the patient rather than gaining something. In other words, the future loss of teeth due to periodontal disease may be more motivating than healthy gums. Once the goal is set, as led and directed by the dentist, based on the patient's mindset and viewpoint, and the patient has been educated on its importance, then discussion may be had to how to obtain it.

On the patient's first visit, which is usually either an emergency or an exam and cleaning, the patient may be given a new patient "goodie" bag with a toothbrush, floss, sample of toothpaste, and an office brochure. A welcome to the practice letter should be sent immediately to the patient with an office brochure and a small handwritten welcome and signed by the doctor. If it was an emergency, a small handwritten note written by the doctor hoping they feel better should be added to the welcome letter. If they were referred, a thank you letter should be sent to the referral person with a small token of appreciation such as a $1.00 lottery ticket. Many states and codes of ethics make it unlawful or unacceptable to actually pay for referrals. But a $1.00 scratch-off lottery ticket is less than a cup of coffee and is no way enough to coerce a referral. It is just being nice and thankful.

This is all being done to communicate to the patient that your office is taking the leadership in their dental care. It also shows that you and your staff will be working with them to obtain their dental goals.

Simply knowing what a goal is does not make it obtainable. In the dental office, patients may want a goal but cannot see how to obtain it. There are many obstacles, but fear, finances, and time are the most common. It is through good listening and educational discussion that the dentist will begin to understand the patient's hurdle to accepting proposed treatment.

References

1 Mehrabian, A. Silent Messages: Implicit Communication of Emotions and Attitudes. 2nd ed. Wadsworth, Belmont, CA; 1981.

2 Ledlow, G.R. and Coppola, M.N. (2011). Leadership for Health Professionals, 120. Sudbury, MA: Jones and Bartlett Learning.

3 Corah, N., Oshea, R., Bissell, G. et al. (1988). The dentist-patient relationship: perceived dentist behaviors that reduce patient anxiety and increase satisfaction. *The Journal of the American Dental Association* 116: 73–76. p 153-cite 110.

4 Young, L.B., O'Toole, C., and Wolf, B. (2015). Communication Skills for Dental Health Care Providers, 141–145. Chicago, IL: Quintessence Publishing.

5 Young, L.B., O'Toole, C., and Wolf, B. (2015). Communication Skills for Dental Health Care Providers, 73. Hanover Park, IL: Quintessence Publishing.

6 Young, L.B., O'Toole, C., and Wolf, B. (2015). Communication Skills for Dental Health Care Providers, 75. Hanover Park, IL: Quintessence Publishing.

7 Graskemper, J. (2011). Professional Responsibility in Dentistry: A Practical Guide to Law and Ethics, 166. Ames, IA: Wiley-Blackwell.

8 Ledlow, G.R. and Coppola, M.N. (2011). Leadership for Health Professionals, 131. Sudbury, MA: Jones and Bartlett Learning.

9 Graskemper, J. (2011). Professional Responsibility in Dentistry: A Practical Guide to Law and Ethics, 167. Ames, IA: Wiley-Blackwell.

10 Deems, D. (2016). Lending an ear. *AGD Impact* (July 2016), p. 13.

11 Young, L.B., O'Toole, C., and Wolf, B. (2015). Communication Skills for Dental Health Care Providers, 81. Hanover Park, IL: Quintessence Publishing.

12 Graskemper, J. (2011). Professional Responsibility in Dentistry: A Practical Guide to Law and Ethics, 81. Ames, IA: Wiley-Blackwell.

8

Patient Motivation

> *You miss 100% of the shots you never take.*
> **Wayne Gretzky**

> *There is little difference in people,*
> *but that little difference makes a big difference.*
> *The little difference is attitude.*
> *The big difference is whether it is positive or not.*
> **Napoleon Hill**

Patient motivation is key to a growing successful practice. Having included the patient by involving them through "co-diagnosing" and educating them through "backward diagnosing," you must get the patient motivated to follow through on your proposed treatment plan. Patient motivation begins with you. The healthcare field demands that patient outcomes are of a higher importance than profits. Patients will notice when their care is motivated by your want of profits rather than their treatment outcomes. Every patient outcome may not produce a profit, but the only way to profits is through patient care. Therefore, positive treatment outcomes are of utmost importance to the patient whether you make a profit or not. Some cases just take more time, effort, and expenses than initially planned. Patients look to you to lead them to better oral health. The only way to lead/guide the patient to proper decision making is by involving the patient in the understanding of any viable options, which may have been adapted to the patient's "Dental IQ" and financial abilities, in the evaluation, consideration, and implementation of the treatment plan. You must always be enthusiastic about the treatment plan you are proposing and enthusiastic for the patient in their choice to follow through on your recommendations. Hence, you must love what you do.

Before even attempting to motivate the patient, you need to understand any obstacle preventing the patient from immediate agreement. There are many obstacles for patients, some of which may not even be financially or dentally

Leadership and Communication in Dentistry, First Edition. Joseph P. Graskemper.
© 2019 John Wiley & Sons, Inc. Published 2019 by John Wiley & Sons, Inc.

related. The three major obstacles I have found are fear, finances, and time. Having been part of a phobia clinic for many years, I have found that if fear is the obstacle, you need to find out what the fear is based on. Some of the more common fears are pain during and/or after treatment, needles, and swallowing something. When treating a phobic patient, it takes time and effort on your part to find what exactly the fear is. Each fear takes extra time to understand the exact fear to allow you to dismantle it. The patient's trust becomes unequivocal as you gain an understanding of the patient's fear, address it, and obliviate it. Each of these fears can be easily addressed. In building a trusting doctor–patient relationship by taking the time to properly listen to the patient, most fears can be dismantled because of the patient's newfound trust in the dentist.

True Case (21)

The patient's husband asked the dentist if he treated phobic patients. When the dentist affirmed that he did, the patient asked if he would see his wife who has been receiving general anesthesia for every appointment, even a simple cleaning. The first appointment with the patient's wife was merely meeting the patient in the reception area and a tour of the office. The second appointment was to sit in the dental chair and just discuss her fear. Her fear was pain of the injection and feeling pain during treatment all based on prior bad experiences. Radiographs were taken and an examination at the second appointment. The next appointment was the prophy. The dentist prescribed Xanax and administered nitrous oxide. Although the patient was very nervous and needed a few breaks during the prophy, it ended successfully. The patient now three years later has no use for Xanax or nitrous oxide, even for restorative care including crowns and restoration of implants. Surgery and implant placement were still under general anesthesia.

Although the first couple of appointments and the first couple of years of dental care took twice the normal amount of time, the patient has become a model patient with extreme trust in the dentist and the entire staff. It was time well spent. The patient became a "missionary" preaching how the dentist and staff had patience and took the time to care for her. Slowing down your routine speed for treating phobic patients is the number 1 thing that needs to be done to overcome obstacles of fear and then spend that time properly listening to the patient.

For fear of the needle, you need to find out if it is due to the actual needle, the perceived pain associated with the injection, or something other. To address any of these fears, you must listen and answer the patient clearly to distinguish the fear with empathy and understanding. There are many methods to give a pain-free injection: use topical, shake the area vigorously, and use the smallest gauge needle possible.

True Case (Example) (22)
For those patients afraid of the injection, I have found that explaining what they will feel helps relieve some of the anxiety. I ask them if I can show them by taking their hand and telling them they will feel a small pinch like this. (I give a small pinch on the back of their hand.) Then you will feel pressure like this. (I then press the area I just pinched.) You will also feel me shaking the area vigorously.

For the fear of swallowing something, simply use a rubber dam, if possible, throat pack, or even practice with the patient and assistant to show the patient how well the high-volume suction works. Also sitting the patient in a more upright position may help. It only takes a few more minutes to do this tell-show-do. The patient will most times feel reassured that you and the assistant are aware of anything possibly being swallowed. This extra time and effort spent is well spent in allowing the patient to endure dental treatment more comfortably. It also encourages the patient to continue with current dental needs and future follow-through with properly scheduled maintenance and re-care visits.

Fear of pain at the time of treatment and after treatment is also very common. With such a patient, before you even begin to treat, explain that the patient is in control and whenever they need a break, feeling uncomfortable, or something is hurting to raise their hand and you will stop immediately and take care of their concern. It is important to ask many times during the procedure, even before the patient raises their hand if they are comfortable. To impress upon the patient that you are not just saying it, once you begin the procedure, simply stop and say, "I thought I saw you raise your hand slightly, is everything ok?" This reassures the patient that you and your assistant are being attentive to their fears and needs.

Regarding fear after the dental visit, your response should vary with the intensity of the treatment you provided and the extent of the patient's fears. It is always advisable to call the patient in the evening of the day of treatment to see how they are doing, especially with any invasive procedure such as endo-dontics or surgery. Even giving the patient your cellphone number gives them the feeling of security if they need you. I have given out my personal cellphone number to patients following invasive procedures, highly stressed, fearful patients, and those I feel need a "security blanket." In over 40 years of practice, I have been called less than five times regarding after treatment concerns. The one minute evening phone call after treatment, when needed, is done on your time and heads off the unexpected patient phone call. It also gives the patient further reassurance of your professional care. Many times, you only get to leave a message. For example, after an extraction, "Just calling to make sure all is OK and that the bleeding has stopped and you are comfortable. There is no need to call me back unless you are having a problem. See you at your next visit."

This is not only a great practice builder but an excellent risk management. Many patients often say they never had a dentist call after their appointment to see how they were doing. It really makes an impression upon them. It also allows you to be on top of any posttreatment problems while they are small and easily remedied, rather than waiting till the patient realizes they have a big problem.

Finances are often a hurdle for the patient even if they have dental insurance. There are many ways to finance treatment, which is beyond the scope of this book. But what is necessary is how you present the need for payment. Many have set aside a separate room to communicate and discuss the proposed treatment with the staff person often titled finance coordinator or insurance coordinator at another appointment. Others believe discussion with the patient is best done chairside at the time of examination. I have found that discussion chairside is best because the patient is already somewhat motivated since they made the appointment and showed up. Making another appointment just gives time for the patient to move his or her attention on to something else. Life happens and as time passes till a consult appointment, the patient's want to get dental care wanes and the dental dollar is spent elsewhere. When communicating the financial component with the patient, you must understand that the money spent is discretionary, unless pain or aesthetics drives the patient to seek care. By discussing finances chairside, you and a staff person are able to elevate that initial motivation of the patient's need immediately into a want of a goal. Most patients have very busy lives and their time is as valuable as yours. Of course, the more complex treatment plan may necessitate a second consultation visit for patient education of the proposed treatment plan options. The patient most likely will boil it all down to two questions:

1) Do I need/value this care?
2) Can I fit this care into my budget and schedule?

True Case (23)

A young dentist, having a very busy day, was falling behind on schedule. One of the patients, which had to wait an hour, was quite upset. The patient was a highly noted attorney who saw time as money. He explained this to the young dentist that waiting an hour, he lost $600.00, which was his fee per hour, and could have been working in his office and come an hour later. He then explained to this young dentist that regardless of the patient, everyone's time is just as important as the dentist's. Patients should be informed of the schedule being off and given the option to wait and/or the opportunity to reschedule. The young dentist took the advice and became noted thereafter as always being on time! A true practice builder.

There are also many views on the issue of who in the office should communicate and discuss finances with the patient. It is best to have a staff member to talk to the patient regarding finances because when the dentist does it, the patient can put the dentist into a dilemma. If the patient asks for a discount, a courtesy, and/or payment over time, the dentist is put into the situation that if he or she refuses, it may appear to the patient that the dentist only cares about the money and not the needs of the patient. Most dentists being caring and having the need of maintaining the patient's trust in them will allow to varying degrees the patient's requests so they do not appear to only care about the finances. Therefore, it is best to have the staff discuss finances so the dentist is not put into the finances versus care discussion. If your office participates in insurance, there is also the issue of the many different insurance policies and fee schedules that must be taken into account in financial discussions.

There are also outside third-party patient financing such as CareCredit, iCare, Lending Club, and Citi Health Card. (For more information see chapter 22, *Professional Responsibility in Dentistry*.) Another option is to make your own financial plan adhering to the Federal Truth in Lending Act [1]. Accepting all major credit and debit cards is also an easy way to allow patient to finance their treatment. The production of the practice is also affected when the dentist takes the time to become part of the financial discussion when he or she could be in another operatory treating another patient.

Due to the cost of dental care and the limitations insurance companies place on dental care coverage, many patients need to space out the treatment and/or the payments. To make these obstacles into simple hurdles, you must prioritize the treatment in a mutually agreeable manner. You may need to expand the treatment time to allow for slower completion and better patient follow-through because of personal financial limitations or the amount of time the patient can take out of his or her schedule to complete the treatment plan. Some patients only care about the aesthetics of their smile and not the moderate periodontal disease around the posterior teeth. The dentist needs to remind/reeducate the patient of the end result of having a healthy mouth with a great smile!

The treatment plan should be prioritized into four categories: pain, infection, function, and aesthetics. Of course, there are times when these categories intermingle and must be considered equally at the time of treatment [2]. During a phased-out treatment plan, these four categories may need to be revisited as time passes and new insurance, financial, or new dental issues arise.

For those without insurance, you can offer your own discounted dental fee schedule to help those who need it to obtain the dental care they need. For example, you give a 20% discount from your UCR fee, two cleanings and one full set of radiographs for $275 (which should be close to the cost of a new patient exam, full mouth radiographs and simple prophylaxis). Hence, you are giving the patient a free prophy and an incentive to complete all the treatment proposed. Insurance fees are usually a lot more discounted than 20%, and you have to get pre-authorizations and sometime wait months for payment. Be sure to check your jurisdiction if such a plan is allowed.

The first two obstacles, fear and finances, may be equally hard to work through, but the third main obstacle is normally easier. With patients working harder and longer, just like dentists (just not longer days but also longer time till retirement), finding the time to go to the dentist is not always that easy. To maintain a successful practice, you should have office hours that accommodate the patients to some degree. When I started out over 40 years ago, I had office hours that included two evenings a week and three Saturdays a month. This accommodated almost all patients to appoint at a time convenient to their schedules.

But to truly motivate a patient after overcoming the obvious hurdles just mentioned, you must reach out and connect with the patient. Motivation has four pillars: a goal, knowledge, attitude, and value (as mentioned in Chapter 7) [3].

These four pillars can be seen in intrinsic and extrinsic motivators that control how the patient seeks care [4]. Intrinsic motivators are those that the patient places on themselves to have the desire to seek dental care. Some obvious intrinsic motivators are to be free of pain, to have a better self-image, to be able to chew food, and a concern for systemic health. Each of these is self-motivating for the patient to accept their need for dental care. Extrinsic motivators are those that friends, family, or even society places on the individual to seek dental care. Obvious extrinsic motivators are to have a better smile for social acceptance, eat without embarrassment, and costs of dental care to be fair and reasonable from the patient's point of view. Each of these will motivate the patient to do something dentally to be more acceptable to friends, family, and society in general.

The dentist's goal is obviously to improve the patient's oral health. But what is the patient's goal? To get out of pain? To make their smile better? To take away the sensitivity? All these could be the patent's goal, which has nothing to do with the crown that is needed on an asymptomatic slightly fractured tooth. Address the patient's concern first before moving forward to discuss the more needed care. This may only entail educating the patient regarding the cause of their concern and fulfilling their need to understand that their concern is noted but is not of immediate need and then moving forward with any other discussion of dental care needed to prevent patient harm or pain. This will build trust in the doctor–patient relationship by showing your care and concern for the patient. Once the appropriate goal is presented to the patient, the dentist must then redirect the patient's perceived goal to the dentally needed goal. This is done by educating the patient. But as a goal is reached, such as getting out of pain, a new attainable goal must be placed to lead the patient to better oral health. Once the pain is relieved, then a goal of complete oral health by completing needed restorative and periodontal needs, followed by a goal of maintenance and preservation of oral health. Therefore, the patient's "Dental IQ" is raised to a better understanding of their long-term goals.

With the high-tech tools of full screen images, patient education videos, and educational models available, the patient can easily be given knowledge and educated about their needs. By following your recommendation, the patient will fulfill their perceived goal or need. This most definitely takes time and effort by the whole staff through listening and connecting with the patient on all levels – the front office staff and the back office staff.

Attitude is a little harder. A patient's attitude regarding dental care may be deeply rooted in poor information, bad past experiences, cultural perception of dentistry, and many other things. Take time and be understanding of the patient's life situation or dental viewpoint. To fully understand the patient, you will empower them to do the best care they believe in and can afford. To empower the patient is to match the patient's knowledge and abilities to the task of proper dental care. This is done by understanding the intrinsic and extrinsic motivators affecting the patient. Attitude is also affected by the patient feeling connected with the dentist and staff. Always try to find something to have in common with the patient so there is a connection that allows a feeling of being part of the practice family. There are so many areas of interest that may cross between two people: sports, children, community events, hobbies, travels, and even the weather.

True Case (24)

A new patient came in for a maintenance/re-care appointment, and it was discovered that they had several carious teeth in need of restoration. At the end of the visit, she asked about the lines in her front teeth. Upon examination, the dentist told her that they were stress lines in her teeth and although they were noticeable in certain lighting, they posed no immediate problem. The patient was then educated about possible need of a night guard and be aware of biting in very hard foods. The patient said that was her main concern for coming in, and she now understood that her teeth can have stress just like her brain has stress. She then went on to ask questions on how she could reduce the stress in her teeth.

In motivating the patient, you must find out what the patient perceives is a healthy mouth, and if that perception is correct. Once you connect with the patient by finding a common understanding, that commonness should be outside of dentistry such as having kids, hobbies, sports, or even just the weather. Get to know the patient as if they were your friend. Try to find something that you and the patient agree upon and then build from there. In attempting to find that commonness, do not prejudge the patient's financial abilities or "Dental IQ." What is important is that you connect with the patient whereby the patient builds trust in you and your practice and agrees to use his or her discretionary dollars for dental care.

The entire staff must also make these connections because the patient may place value on only a certain portion of the services you render. The patient may put more value on the fact that you take their insurance or that you will become an advocate for the patient by writing a short narrative for the patient to get the benefits they deserve. Once the patient places value on your service, whether it is front or back office staff services, the patient's attitude will change to achieve the goals you have presented.

As a summary, communication with the patient must:

1) Be the foundation of a trusting doctor–patient relationship.
2) Not be condescending, controlling, or overbearing with the patient.
3) Not be one-way thinking of it "being the doctor's way or no way."
4) Provide an avenue for feedback that may be shaded with the patient's cultural dental beliefs.
5) Be aware of the patient's viewpoint of dentistry.
6) Be flexible and understanding of the patient.
7) Engage the patient to feel included in the treatment plan decisions.
8) Be truthful, honest, and sincere.
9) Be ethical and knowledgeable.
10) Be clear and understanding.
11) Have entire staff embrace the communication effort.

References

1 Graskemper, J. (2011). *Professional Responsibility in Dentistry: A Practical Guide to Law and Ethics*, 168. Ames, IA: Wiley-Blackwell.
2 Graskemper, J. (2011). *Professional Responsibility in Dentistry: A Practical Guide to Law and Ethics*, 101. Ames, IA: Wiley-Blackwell.
3 Beltiz, J. (1991). *Success: Full Living*, 20. The Franciscan Hermitage.
4 Ledlow, G.R. and Coppola, M.N. (2011). *Leadership for Health Professionals*, 113. Sudbury, MA: Jones and Bartlett Learning.

Part II: Your Staff

9

Leadership of Personnel

If your actions inspire others to dream more, learn more and become more, you are a leader.
John Quincy Adams

Surround yourself with the best people you can find, delegate authority and don't interfere.
Ronald Reagan

Your staff is the most crucial component in having a successful practice. Leadership of staff is not like leadership in an organization. Organizations do not depend on their leadership for continued existence. They rely on its membership. Many organizations can withstand and continue to exist even when there is poor leadership for a couple of years. This does not hold true for the dental practice. You may want to view this situation in a manner that you equate patients to membership, but that also does not hold true. Membership pays money to become a member. A patient pays money for a service and staff stays if treated fairly. Therefore, a practice with poor leadership will not grow. It will eventually become non-sustainable if patients and staff do not have leadership. Leading your staff is perhaps the most important role you have to obtain success for your practice. Your staff is the first contact point for a new patient. They are also the conduit to the finances of the practice since they bill and collect from patients and insurance companies. For the practice to run successfully, it is dependent on the staff to reach goals, keep commitments, and be held accountable. It all starts with the hiring of the right staff.

Attracting the right applicants begins with a good ad detailing your needs. Whether it is for a front office receptionist, dental assistant, or dental hygienist job, make the ad inviting to the type of person you want. The new employee should fit your personality but also complement the rest of the staff. You need a mixture of people to have a successful practice.

Leadership and Communication in Dentistry, First Edition. Joseph P. Graskemper.
© 2019 John Wiley & Sons, Inc. Published 2019 by John Wiley & Sons, Inc.

The mixture of employees' various workplace attitudes can be broken down to different methods of working. There are also many viewpoints on how to get everybody on the dental canoe into the right seat – all paddling in the right direction.

In *Professional Responsibility in Dentistry: A Practical Guide To Law and Ethics*, I discussed a simple way of evaluating employees in relationship to various animal intuitive behaviors: bear, owl, rabbit, deer, and monkey [1]. A fun way of getting the right mix of people to work together! There are other assessments available.

The Seven C's is another assessment of a new employee that works best during the 90-day probationary/tryout time. Normally the true person does not really show up till at least a full month has past. By sailing through the Seven "C's," you will see if the new employee will have what it takes to make your team:

- Confident (initiative) – Does the new employee take initiative and goes about their tasks without being asked or told what to do when the employee should already know?
- Comforting (empathy) – Does he or she show empathy toward the patient when needed?
- Caring (understanding) – Is the person a good listener for the patient, showing his or her understanding of the patient's needs?
- Competent (knowledgeable) – Do they know their stuff?
- Cleanliness (knows what clean means) – Are they thorough in their cleaning of the operatory, instruments, and personal appearance?
- Cheerful (happy to be there) – Do they have a positive outlook on life and appreciative of being part of your dental team?
- Courtesy (respectful) – Does the new employee show respect and friendliness to patient, staff, and you, the owner? [1]

The Kolbe Assessment looks at how a person naturally operates. It is how you get things done when you have the freedom to do it your way – your instinctive way of approaching and solving difficult problems. It is based on the cognitive, affective, and conative levels of effort. Cognitive and affective efforts are generally understood. But what is conative? It is a conscious effort to carry out self-determined acts [2]. It is your natural tendencies and impulses that direct your actions. A full discussion is beyond the scope of this book, but Kolbe can be broken down to four areas:

Fact Finder – How you gather information and share it (lots of questions, yelps, googles, researches before making a decision).
Follow Through – The way you arrange and design (lots of lists, OCD?, highly organized closet).
Quick Start – How you deal with risk and uncertainty (trying new things without hesitation, able to improvise on the spot, visionary).

Implementor – How you handle space and tangibles (read people well, able to fix things around the house, able to build things from scratch) [3].

Another assessment available is ADEA (Analytical, Driver, Amiable, and Expressive):

1) Analytical

One who asks questions to gather data, information, and insights to guide direction and decisions.

The analytical personality type is very deep and thoughtful. They're serious and purposeful individuals. They set very high standards, so they have very high standards of performance personally and professionally. Analyticals are orderly and organized. They also tend to have that really dry but witty sense of humor.

Analytical strengths are that they are perfectionists. They want things done right and they want them done right the first time. They're neat and tidy individuals. Analyticals are economical, and they are self-disciplined.

Analyticals' weaknesses are that they can be moody, critical, and negative. Analyticals can be indecisive and they overanalyze everything. Their perfectionism can also manifest as a weakness at times, as they can be guilty of making their pursuit of perfection stall completion.

2) Driver

One who likes to be in charge and have a say in the control of a situation – usually a very energetic person who likes to be "in" on it and get others to follow.

Drivers are the dynamic and active personality type. They exude confidence and naturally gravitate toward leadership positions. They move very quickly to action, but they are not detail oriented. Drivers are great with the big picture – they're visionaries and they see how we're going to get to where we need to go, but they're not always great at taking the interim steps needed to get there.

You can probably see how an analytical and a driver might not work very well together – but also that their skills can nicely complement each other. It can be said that if you want to get to the moon, you hire a driver, but if you want to get back, you hire an analytical.

Drivers' strengths are that they are very determined individuals. They are independent and they are productive. Drivers get a lot of things done. They are visionaries and they're decisive. A driver would rather make a bad decision than no decision. They just want that decision to be made.

On the weak side, the driver can be insensitive, unsympathetic, harsh, proud, and sarcastic. Drivers do not like to admit when they are wrong. They can also rush to a decision without thoroughly thinking through or understanding the results or consequences of their decision.

3) Amiable

One who shows their feelings freely – usually very friendly, likeable by all, and easily connects to many types of patients.

The amiable personality type is a very patient and well-balanced individual. They're quiet but witty. They're very sympathetic, kind, and inoffensive – amiables do not like to offend people.

An amiable is easy going and everybody likes the amiables. You know why? Because they don't like conflict so they're very easy to get along with. They're diplomatic and calm. But on the weak side, amiables can be stubborn and selfish. Their aversion to offense and conflict can also manifest as a weakness.

4) Expressive

One who is not shy to speak his or her thoughts and suggestions – usually animated in their manner of communication.

We call the expressive the social specialist because they love to have fun. They are individuals who turn disaster into humor, they prevent dull moments, and they are very generous people. They want to be included. Expressives want to be included in projects. They want to be included on teams. They want to be included in conversations.

On the strong side, the expressive is very outgoing. They are ambitious, charismatic, and persuasive. On the weak side, they can be disorganized, undisciplined, loud, and incredibly talkative. Expressives can talk up to 200 words a minute with gusts up to 300. They can talk.

Of course, these are generalizations, and many people will exhibit some amount of any number of these personality types. However, everyone will more strongly exhibit characteristics of one type over all the others. Recognizing and understanding which personality types you are managing on your team will help you motivate and communicate with them [4].

No matter what assessment you use, it has been found that a motivated and inspired employee is your best bet. Motivation is all about getting a person to start and persist on a task or project. Inspiration is the emotive feeling of value a person experiences while performing a worthy task or project. Those with high motivation and inspiration in their jobs often become team leaders [5].

The patients are all different, so you need to have various types of staff members to relate to all the patients. This provides a personal touch for the patient when he or she wants a specific staff member for hygiene or to follow through on an insurance claim because of a perceived special connection to that staff member. Once you have in your mind the type of person that you would like to hire, you then need to start with a decent ad.

"Dental assistant needed call (123-456-7890)" will not attract the best applicants. For example, "Dental Assistant needed full time in Jones Village. Must be energetic, positive, have initiative, and a 2 year minimum experience to join growing dental team. Call (office phone number for an interview, fax resume to _____ or email resume' to _____)" is a better approach and will attract more applicants [6]. There are many places for the ad to appear such as Craigslist, Indeed, and local newspapers.

After reviewing the various resumes, you will need to meet with the applicant. You may either do this yourself or delegate an initial interview with a staff member, if you trust that individual's interviewing skills. The interview should have open-ended questions to allow the applicant to talk. Besides asking about dental job experiences, also ask about hobbies and other things that would allow the applicant to talk about themselves so you may get an idea of whether he or she is the one to hire. Try and learn as much about the person as possible since they will become a vital member of your dental team. The main question is: "Will you be able to work with this person?" Some good examples could be:

Tell me about a time where you had to use patience to calm a patient down.
Have you ever been at odds with a coworker? How did you handle it?
Describe a goal you set for your self and how you met it.
How do you handle interruptions?
Describe what customer service means to you.
What five words best describe you?

Make sure their handwriting is acceptable especially if working in the front desk area by having them write a short sentence. Check references by contacting the former employer. There is really only one question that matters in your inquiry: "Would you hire him/her again?" If the reference source would not hire the applicant again, then it would be wise not to hire the applicant. If you decide to continue your search, I have found that usually the best choices are within the first three interviewees. Unless there are many good candidates available, the chances of finding anyone better are lessened as time passes. This is because a motivated applicant is not going to wait for the job. They want and/or need the job immediately and are motivated to do so.

Once you have decided to hire the person, it is best to have a working interview for a day or 2. Law requires you to pay the applicant for the working interview. This allows the employer and the entire staff to see if he or she is a good match for the practice. After the working interview, showing your trust in the team you have developed, you should ask what the other team members honestly think of the applicant. Remember besides your self, they are the ones who have to work side and side with the new employee. This also gives the employees a sense of ownership in the team culture you are creating. Then, if your decision was correct, you then need to inform the person of employment and have them read and sign the office policy manual that will be covered in the next chapter.

It is the practice's culture you are trying to cultivate in this new employee and successfully incorporate him or her into your practice. It is the practice's culture that holds the team bonded together to make a successful practice great.

An organization's culture is the pattern of basic assumptions discovered or developed by a given group (staff) or as it learns to cope with its problems of external adaptation and integration; these assumptions have worked well enough to be considered valid and therefore are taught to new members as the correct way to perceive, think, or feel in relations to their mutual office problems, challenges, and opportunities [7], or simply stated: "Important understandings (often unstated) that members of a community share in common" [8]. It is important that the entire staff shares your mission to accomplish your vision. By having the staff give their input on a possible future coworker, they have a stake in his or her success and that of the office. It is the staff that many times will look out for you and the practice when the unexpected happens.

Once you have made your decision to hire an applicant, they should be on a 90-day tryout period. Don't be afraid that if you think you have a diamond in the rough and the 90-day tryout needs to be extended. Many times a new employee, especially one without experience, realizes they need more time to feel they belong and feel "in" on the office culture. I recommend you do so for the right person. According to Jay Grier there are basically seven steps to hiring the right person that can be applied during the 90-day tryout period:

1) Check out the ATTITUDE!
2) What are their experiences? (Ask about an unique experience and how it affected them.)
3) Assessments – try to categorize over the 90-day tryout (use Seven C's, Kolbe, and/or ADEA).
4) Match skills and talent to the needed position that fits to you and your staff.
5) Educate and acclimate the person to your practice's culture. See if they want "IN."
6) Do they get "IT"?? Are they incorporated into the practice during the 90 days, or are they a loaner?
7) Continuous encouragement, track progress, and manage to highest personal potential [9].

True Case (25)

A recently new employee started to always point out what was wrong and how it was done at her previous office. This new employee would point out how fellow employees were doing it wrong or not like it should be done when the dentist was not around. The rest of the staff started to resent the coworker and often told the dentist that he needed to get rid of this new employee. Finally, at the monthly office meeting, she started to say how things should change and be done her way. The dentist then asked the employee to walk with him outside the front door and asked her whose name is on top of the other four dentists. She said, "You are." He said, "You're right and you're fired." He then proceeded to escort her to her locker to gather her things and leave.

If the person you hired is found not to be a good fit for your practice, you must let that person go immediately to find a better employment opportunity elsewhere and begin the employee search again. A bad employee could poison an entire staff quicker than you think.

It is important to fire the person in a professional manner. Do not become angry or emotional about the firing. Always have a witness when you do fire an employee. Prior to firing an employee regardless of how long they were employed, you must maintain an employment file on each employee individually. As the situation arises, documentation of the problem is a must. To properly fire an employee, the problem must be documented several times unless it is so outrageous as to legality or patient safety. You need to give guidance to correct the unwanted behavior, which is usually the first warning that is verbal and should be documented in the employee's record. It should also be noted what was told to the employee to remedy the situation. Then, the second warning, which should be written with what is wrong and how to correct it, is signed by the employee and witnessed. The third notice, which is also written, is the dismissal/termination of the employee for the stated reason and again should be signed by the employee and a witness [10]. Examples are continued tardiness, not cleaning the operatory properly, not wearing or not properly utilizing universal/standard precautions, etc. The problem should also be a repeated offense, unless of course it is serious enough to warrant immediate termination as pointed out in the office policy manual. It helps to have written employee warnings that the employee also signs so there will be no miscommunication. When there is enough evidence to allow you to fire the employee, do so. Try not to base the firing on your emotions.

True Case (26)

An employee of many years started to act little differently for about a month prior. This employee of eight years had grown into one of the dental team leaders. The dentist had been through the employee's boyfriend breakups, a pregnancy, a marriage, and now another pregnancy. The employee has been complaining to coworkers and the dentist that she did not know how she was going to pay for childcare for two children both under the age of 3. She started to tell the dentist that he was rude and mean to staff and patients. She started to come in late and not be a team player as she had been the past eight years. One day the dentist asked privately what the problem was since it was not like her to be so. She immediately asked, "Are you firing me?" The dentist replied, "No, just what is the problem." She yelled so all could hear, "You're firing me, right?" He said, "No, why don't you leave and take a break for a while." She then yelled, "Your firing me?" The dentist by this time also quite irate said, "You want to be fired – You're fired!" The employee gathered her things and left smiling out the front door. She had the baby two weeks later and unemployment for support.

In cases when you, as the leader, feel that it is better to work with the underperforming employee, then you should make the endeavor if it is better for the practice in the long run. In trying to reverse an underperforming employee, you must look to the possible reasons for their unacceptable job performance:

1) Are there possible unexpected and unshared personal problems?
2) Does employee not feel valued or appreciated by you or someone else on the dental team?
3) Was the employee properly trained and/or told what was expected and is now frustrated with job duties?
4) Does the employee see the job as a dead end personally and/or professionally?

It is my belief that if the offense is minor and the employee is truly trying to improve or remedy the situation, it is always better to work with someone you already know a little about than start off from the beginning again. A constructive meeting is needed immediately as soon as the performance of an employee waivers from the expected. The longer this meeting is put off, the worse the problem becomes and the larger the negative impact on the practice. Even with patience and constant effort to turn an underperforming employee into a contributing member of the dental team, you never know what kind of person you will get the next time around. It could be worse.

True Case (27)

A dentist with a very successful team-oriented practice was in need of a new assistant. Deciding on hiring a newly graduated dental assistant from a dental assistant school, he envisioned training the newly minted dental assistant to become the best assistant he would ever have. After three months of attempting to train her, he decided that is was not working out. An opening in the front office was occurring at the same time. The dental assistant was a great fit for the team in all aspects except the specific job duties she was hired for. She had a great understanding of people, is respectful of the patients, and got along with the entire staff. So, he moved her to the front desk to greet patients, make appointments, and learn insurance coding and billing. A few years later, the person doing the insurance billing for 10 years retired. Again, the dentist needed a new employee. He again moved the employee into the main insurance billing position and hired a new employee for the front desk. He was hesitant to do so because the employee hadn't shown much understanding of the insurance but wished to stick with someone he knew rather than hire an unknown for such a critical job. To his surprise she turned out to be the best person for that position. She finally felt "in" and accomplished more than expected by the dentist and the employee.

Choosing your staff is probably one of the most important duties of the dentist because the successful dentist will delegate many job duties to the staff. They will indirectly be in control of the finances of the practice from arranging patient finances and payments, including proper insurance coverage and payments, to ordering office and dental supplies. The success of delegation depends on the quality of staff hired and the communication skills of the dentist. That communication starts with all individual staff members knowing their job duties and what is expected of them. They must also be given the tools necessary to accomplish their job. Merely delegating to the staff is not leadership that will allow the practice to achieve its goals. To successfully lead the practice, the dentist must constantly be enthusiastic and focused on practice improvement.

Are you forming a group or a team? A group is two or more individuals who come from random disciplines (front and back office duties) with no apparent collective skills (one cannot work without the other) to accomplish complex and specific tasks (run a practice from assisting surgery to understanding insurance coding). However a team is an interdisciplinary group of individuals who are brought together to accomplish specific tasks or projects and to work together for the success of the collective group, your practice [11]. Great leadership turns a group into a team.

To turn a group into a team, all members must develop a close positive group affiliation whereby the group will collectively adapt, buy into, and embrace the practice culture, goals, and success. Staff members will move beyond their own self-interests to focus more on larger mutual interests – the practice. Over time, the team will take ownership, along with the dentist leader, of the practice culture. This is done by allowing some inclusion to all staff as is warranted, giving some control to staff members, holding them accountable, and making all feel wanted and needed. To build the team all must have a mutual work ethic that supports the practice's mission and value statements. As the new hire becomes familiarized with the entire existing team, they will be transforming from being a "coached" member who usually consider themselves as "out" to a "mentored" member who considers themselves "in." Coaching uses a transformational leadership style since you are trying to shape and inspire the new employee to fit into your team. Coaching a new employee is done not just by the dentist but by the entire team. This entails the entire team to educate the new employee as to their specific job duties, challenging the new employee to keep interest, understanding the practice culture, and obtaining certain individual goals of a new employee to show and feel progress toward being "in." This is true positive energy that makes the whole team vibrant and succeed to make the practice better.

Mentoring is less job specific and more about career building and understanding the practice culture. As an employee moves from coaching level to mentoring level, more is delegated, with more responsibility and accountability, allowing the employee to grow and become more valuable to the practice. This is normally a slow process where the new employee must first walk before running. The staff does not need to be "in" or included in all facets of the practice. How much influence do you want to allow the staff to be affected by such knowledge? To be considered "in," the new employee must understand and appreciate how his or her role/job duties affect the whole team, thereby creating a synergistic team effort that the whole team is motivated and all strive to even go beyond their own expectations. As the dentist leader, you need to tap into the synergistic environment to build a cohesive and productive team that meets the philosophy and goals of the practice. As the team matures and becomes part of the practice by your leadership investment of time and effort, they add to the practice as intellectual capital. The value of the practice is increased by the team's talent and belief in the practice culture. They become empowered and emotionally vested to make the practice the best it can be.

Once you have delegated and made sure the staff member is properly trained and has the tools available to perform the job delegated, you must follow up with the employee and make sure they are accountable. When employees take responsibility for their actions, you will see higher quality and productivity. Are they doing the job well or better than you expected? If not, you must help the employee improve their efforts to fulfill the delegated job. If they do not succeed with improvement to meet your expectations, take the job away from the employee or allow the employee to find better suited employment elsewhere. Although you tried to hire the very best fit for the team you are building, you must remember that there will always be a highly motivated, self-reliant, ever busy "in" group or individual and there will always be the less motivated, do my work and go home "out" group or individual. Understand that all employees, being human, are different and each must be led differently at times, so all feel to be "in," such that the practice receives the full value of the employee's worth. Hence, focus your efforts on building each staff member's strength and not on trying to change the person to overcome their weakness. The practice must receive a return on the employee's training and work.

Keeping a great team motivated also takes some effort from the dentist leader. There are many ways to keep the team motivated. Wages and salaries are not the only motivators. A simple "Good morning" and "Thank you" on a daily basis can make an employee appreciated [12].

There are also many team building seminars available that you can attend with the team. However, if you do not carry through on the presented suggestions, which the team thought were important, it may not work as well as you thought. The expense may have outweighed the outcome.

I suggest some simple things that can be easily done and well appreciated are:

1) Say "Thank you," and mean it, after work each day.
2) Remember their special days (birthdays, anniversaries, children's birthdays).
3) Arrange a social outing (bowling, miniature golf, special lunch, "happy hour").

4) Have a "bravo board" to designate an "employee of the month."
5) Send flowers (or bagels, cake, or fruit basket) to the office.
6) Hand out car wash or restaurant gift certificates, lottery tickets, or lunches.

Feel free to use your imagination! Don't forget the element of surprise [13].

To lead the team together and individually, there are five easy inquiries that need to be made for accountability and for achieving the practice goals as held in the mission and vision statements:

1) What's the plan? What are you trying to achieve?
2) Does the intended goals placed on the team or individual help the practice on any or every level?
3) Are the goals given too lofty and unattainable? Are they understood by all who need to work to achieve the goal?
4) How can you objectively see if progress is made toward the goal?
5) What strategies (guidance) have you the dentist leader put in place to enable the team or individual employee to succeed for the betterment of the practice?

> For example, you want the production to increase (The Plan). Increased production leads to increased profits which allows for possibly higher bonuses or wages (Goals placed). The entire staff should understand the importance and the results of achieving the goal for the team and for the individual employee. It should not be so lofty as to be unattainable. Daily review of the daysheets will reveal if progress is being made toward the goal of increase production. MOST importantly, you must give guidance to the staff on how to achieve the goal and have a successful plan. (Knowledge to achieve goal) (were fees raised, more hours added, front and back office become more efficient, better follow-up on non-completed treatment plans, better follow-up on insurance processing. etc.) As the goals are met, bonuses become more common. (Employee Attitudes change with increased income and places Value on the plan) THE RESULT – A MOTIVATED TEAM!!

After a number of years and having the best team you can have, there will situations that arise causing conflict among individual employees and conflict between the dentist and an employee or the entire staff. It happens and it is unavoidable. It is much like a family, which, at times, has disagreements and/or different opinions. Remember you will eventually have a team that has invested time and effort into your practice and its culture, making your practice the best it can be. This may even necessitate a change in the office policy manual to reflect changes due to a variety of outside influences (loss of patients due to changes of insurance, change in patient demographics, increased competition, etc.)

Conflicts also occur in dealing with different personal cultural understandings and personal versus group issues.

True Cases (28)

An employee of 10 years became very upset because she and the rest of the staff did not get paid when the office was closed due to inclement weather. Being an hourly wage earner, she stated that she was able to come in, but I had closed the office and therefore I should pay her for the day. She stated that her father and her husband both work at large corporations and both were paid when inclement weather occurred. Her "office culture" was that of a large corporation's policies for salaried employees. I explained the differences and though upset she understood.

To help conflict resolution within the staff, you must identify the conflict as soon as possible. Have both employees to meet in your office to narrow down the issue so as to what exactly the issue is. Focus on the mutual interests of the office: know what you are willing to do if conflict is not resolved, know what solution you can live with, and base the result on facts that are objective. As the dentist leader, you must listen equally and fully to each party prior to making a decision as to how to resolve the conflict. Depending on the issues, after hearing both sides, attempt to narrow down the issue as much as possible before making any decision. Conflicts between employees are more common in larger offices due to the fact there are more employees with different viewpoints, mindsets, and life experiences. I have sent both to an early lunch with money to buy each lunch and to have them resolve it during lunch. Usually this results in a positive resolution when the issues are small.

There are six ways to manage conflicts:

1) Be accommodating to both to minimize loss to the practice by working out a solution that all lose a little and gain a little.
2) Avoiding the conflict if it is trivial and has little to negligible impact on the practice. Letting it "blow over."
3) You can at times collaborate with both by merging the issues into one that all can agree upon and getting both to work together to resolve it.
4) If it is a competing conflict in which both are intense in their stances, then an immediate decision must be had. This may necessitate firing an employee.
5) If the conflict does not have a great impact on the practice or does not cause much disruption, then possibly compromising with the employee should be considered.
6) If all parties of the conflict are a little flexible, then a solution should be worked toward to all parties' satisfaction [14].

In building a great dental team, be sure to remember that the entire staff looks to you as a guide. You must lead by example. You never should ask an employee to do something that you are not willing to do your self: from picking up something on the floor to help cleaning instruments or an operatory. With any interaction with an employee, you must not be indecisive or arbitrary. You must be definitive to avoid any miscommunication and to be equal and fair to all.

Some conflicts may result in letting an employee find career opportunities elsewhere. There are seven tips on making the situation of firing as painless as possible:

1) Meet in private and have a witness present. Make no surprises out of it and schedule the meeting when there are no patients.
2) Be clear as to the reason why the employee is being terminated.
3) Don't waste time going into details. Hopefully you have followed the three-step employee warning regarding cause for termination.
4) Don't be defensive if the employee makes accusations or insults. Keep your emotions in check so you are not in an argument with them.
5) Pay the employee. Have their last paycheck and any other benefits owed ready if possible. If not, let them know when they can expect it and then make sure you follow through as promised. Check with your local jurisdiction regarding last paycheck rules and regulations. Some have a time period within which it must be paid.
6) Try to end it on a positive note and wishing them well in any new endeavor. If possible, offer a letter of recommendation.
7) Let the other team members know what has occurred to eliminate speculation and gossip [15].

There are some caveats that must be mentioned. Dentists working in a very confined area tend to become micromanagers, looking at every little facet of the practice. It is important to keep an eye on the entire practice but you have to allow the great individuals you just hired to do their jobs without browbeating or being told how to do every little thing about the job. Demanding an error-free environment is difficult, if not non-attainable, because all are human individuals. We all have that "human moment" of unexpected, unintended mistakes that just happen, even with the best intentions. When this happens, the dentist leader must evaluate and decide on how large the mistake impacts and affects the practice. Some mistakes may lead to termination rather than simple intervention and training. Are you going to micromanage to the point of being a dictator or are you willing to lead a staff with delegated duties? We are all working with humans so errors are unavoidable and should be used to learn and improve the practice. Employees will grow when given autonomy and freedom to fulfill their job duties. Also, allowing input from the team on how to improve the practice is often overlooked by dentists who maintain a paternal/military-like leadership. Many times, the patients will talk to the staff (hygienist, assistants, and front office) about how they feel toward the dentist, or the staff may suggest an improvement on how patients are treated. The staff has a connection to what patients are thinking and saying, sometimes more than the dentist. Listen to the staff's suggestions and consider them as from the patient's point of view. Not all are actionable, but many times the suggestions are truly for the betterment of the practice.

True Case (29)

At the monthly meeting, the staff brought up an issue that several patients were having with the dentist. They stated that the patients feel the dentist is always in a rush and talks too fast such that they don't understand him, and he is gone before they can ask any questions. In other words, the staff told the dentist he needs to slow down and start paying attention to the patients again. Although the dentist's ego was a little hurt, he took their advice, worked on changing his ways, and slowed down. The patient noticed the difference and the practice continued to grow.

Remember as leader/owner of the practice, you must wear the four "hats" that every successful dentist leader must wear to maintain the interconnectedness of the staff:

1) Player – You are working together with the staff. You are not merely being an administrator dictating policies. In a small office especially, you work side by side with your employees providing care for your patients.
2) Coach – You must bring out the best in each team member, give direction, and have them work together for the betterment of all, much like a champion sports team. Each member must know and appreciate what each member contributes.
3) Manager – You must keep the team together and motivated. You must promote the practice for a constant influx of new patients, seek new team members when needed, and maintain a community presence for growth.
4) Owner – You must make sure there is a profit in the end to assure the return of investment of your time, efforts, and finances and provide for capital improvement (new equipment) as needed [16].

Therefore, the mindset of the dentist is very important. Is the dentist leader just:

Doing a filling?
Treating a patent?
Building a practice?
Working to be successful at living?

The mindset of the dentist is what guides the practice and employees. The dentist leader must constantly build the practice and team to become successful at living. Here is another way to look at this most important mindset: Are you a thermometer that merely records the information or are you a thermostat that sets the mood?

Be aware of small bad habits that dentists fall into that detours a dentist from being the best they can be:

1) Procrastination – Not updating your computer software/hardware, not reviewing employee performance in a timely manner, not reviewing your insurance involvement. Do not overanalyze any reasonable changes to move the practice and staff to be the best it can be. Overanalyzing leads to "analysis paralysis" whereby nothing progresses.
2) Impulsiveness – Jumping on the latest trend without thinking it through if it is applicable to your practice, firing a good employee over a small mistake, allowing emotions to guide your business decisions.
3) Complacency – Life changes, times change. Not responding to the changing demographics surrounding your practice and what current and future patients want and expect.
4) Failure to follow through – Making promises to the staff but never delivering undermines your leadership to the point the staff will stop following you [17].

It is very important to not make a very large change in the practice that would affect the team members to minimize non-acceptance and reduce any conflicts that may arise. You want to continually improve the practice through small steps so all may easily accept and implement the change. The Kaizen theory best describes this type of improvement. Small improvements executed continuously have a bigger effect on improvement in quality because small changes are easier to be accepted by staff/patients by becoming slowly imbedded in the practice culture than one big change that shakes the status quo [18].

There are thirteen steps for taking a good team to great team:

1) Starts with superb people. Recruit the best people possible.
2) Great teams and great leaders create one another. Collaboration is critical. Old control leadership models do not work. Great teams are treated decisively and fairly.
3) Every great team has a great leader. A leader is an organizer of genius, who is a pragmatic dreamer and who has an original, yet attainable vision. He or she makes the vision statement a reality.
4) Great team leaders love talent, know where to find it, and revel in the talent of others. They give true appreciation for the talent and skills of individual team members always acknowledging the individual's contribution.
5) Great teams are full of talented people who can work together, sharing information and advancing the practice as the only real social obligation. They use their collective talent to communicate with each other and with patients for the betterment of the practice – sharing is caring.

6) Great teams think they are on a tremendously important mission. They are believers. Their clear, collective purpose makes everything they do seem meaningful and valuable. Each team member must believe what they are doing is a meaningful, valuable part of the practice's mission. They believe in the dentist and the practice.

7) Great teams see themselves as winning underdogs. They will always work with extra effort to have that extra edge to always improve.

8) Great teams are optimistic not settling for realistic status quo. They believe that it can always get better because it will be better – always improving.

9) In great teams, the right person has the right job. Although some cross-training is important, especially for a small office, each must work in the area of their greatest strengths. Getting all the right people in the right seat on the dental team canoe!

10) Great teams are given what they need and are free from meaningless and useless information and materials. They get the necessary instruments and capital improvements needed to improve the practice.

11) Great teams share information effectively. Everyone has full access to any needed information. They believe the necessity to be cross-trained if only for an understanding and appreciation of the other team member's role within the team.

12) Great teams produce. They understand the importance of the end product in dentistry as being a service to improve patient care. The better the service to the patient, the more profitable the practice is.

13) Great work is its own reward. Each team member is intrinsically motivated to do their best for the good of the team. They love their jobs! [19]

There is a level of teaming that is exemplified as an expert team. Many refer to this as the "Dream Team." An expert team is defined as a set of interdependent team members, each of whom possesses unique and expert-level knowledge, skills, and experience related to task performance and who adapt, coordinate, and cooperate as a team, thereby producing sustainable and repeatable team functioning at superior or at least near-optimal level or performance [20]. Expert teams are composed of members who anticipate each other's needs and coordinate their action without necessarily or always engaging in overt communication because they share an experience of tacit communication arising from a shared knowledge of tasks and team processes [21].

To achieve an expert "Dream Team" in a newly acquired or start-up practice where all the employees are new, you must first get all in the "office canoe" facing the right way and not tipping the canoe over. Being a dentist leader, it is up to you to set the practice/office culture through your mission and vision statements. Have all your employees read, understand, and believe in the mission and vision statements. With all new employees, you must start as a coach to get your players/team members to work first as a group. Some employees will do well and quickly find the right seat in the canoe and start paddling in the right direction. Some will not even make it into the canoe and will need to seek employment opportunities elsewhere. As the practice matures, the dentist leader must coach the group the need for cross-training to understand and appreciate the other coworkers' contribution to the team. This takes time and effort by all to achieve and is highly dependent on your leadership. This ensures that the practice continues to operate smoothly even when a group/team member is on vacation or extended sick leave. As the cross-training occurs and the group is molded into a team, the practice/office culture becomes engrained in each team member. They begin to have job duty thought integration whereby all become intrinsically motivated working tacitly to become that Expert Dream Team you hoped for with your leadership.

Even though you try to have all the dental team working together meeting their individual potentials and that of the practice, you may never really know your employees.

True Case (30)

An employee of two years came into the dentist's office and stated that she was offered another dental assisting job for $4.00 more per hour. The dentist not wanting to lose his only assistant agreed to give the assistant a $2.00 an hour raise. She agreed. Two days later she said she needed the $2.00 more an hour and would have to leave if she did not get it. Of course, the dentist offered her the best of luck at her new job and asked if she could hang on for a two weeks' notice. She said no. Two months later, the assistant was on the local news being arrested and accused of multiple robberies that were allegedly drug related. You just never really know!

References

1 Graskemper, J. (2011). *Professional Responsibility in Dentistry: A Practical Guide to Law and Ethics*, 172. Ames, IA: Wiley-Blackwell.
2 Moreno, H. (2016) Kolbe Index – a unique method to assess your talent and improve your quality of your life.
3 Moreno, H. (2018). Kolbe Index – a Unique Method to Assess Your Talent and Improve the Quality of Your Life. www.templatemonster.com/blog/kolbe-index-reveiw/ (accessed 16 December 2018).
4 Fritchen, K. (2015). 4 Personality Types that all Leaders Should Learn to Recognize. http://crestcomleadership.com/2015/11/24/4-personality-types-that-all-leaders-should-learn-to-recognize/ (accessed 16 December 2018).
5 Ledlow and Coppola (2011). *Leadership for Health Professionals*, 113. Sudbury, MA: Jones and Bartlett Learning.

6 Graskemper, J. (2011). *Professional Responsibility in Dentistry: A Practical Guide to Law and Ethics*, 171. Ames, IA: Wiley-Blackwell.

7 (a) Ledlow and Coppola (2011). *Leadership for Health Professionals*, 130. Sudbury, MA: Jones and Bartlett Learning. (b) Schein, E.H. (1999). *The Corporate Culture Survival Guide: Sense and Nonsense About Culture Change*. San Francisco, CA: Jossey-Bass.

8 (a) Ledlow and Coppola (2011). *Leadership for Health Professionals*, 231. Sudbury, MA: Jones and Bartlett Learning. (b) Sathe, V. *Culture and Related Corporate Realities: Text, Cases, and Reading on Organizational Entry, Establishment and Change*, 6. Homewood, IL: Irwin.

9 Grier, J. 7 Steps to hiring the right person, *Dentaltown* (August 2017).

10 Graskemper, J. (2011). *Professional Responsibility in Dentistry: A Practical Guide to Law and Ethics*, 106, 107. Ames, IA: Wiley-Blackwell.

11 Ledlow and Coppola (2011). *Leadership for Health Professionals*, 166. Sudbury, MA: Jones and Bartlett Learning.

12 Blanchard, K. and Johnson, S. (1982). *The One Minute Manager*, 44. New York: Berkley Books.

13 Graskemper, J. (2011). *Professional Responsibility in Dentistry: A Practical Guide to Law and Ethics*, 176. Ames, IA: Wiley-Blackwell.

14 Ledlow and Coppola (2011). *Leadership for Health Professionals*, 126. Sudbury, MA: Jones and Bartlett Learning.

15 McKenzie, S. (2017). 7 Tips on what to do when it's time to fire an employee. www.drbicuspid.com/index (accessed 9 March 2017).

16 Graskemper, J. (2011). *Professional Responsibility in Dentistry: A Practical Guide to Law and Ethics*, 174. Ames, IA: Wiley-Blackwell.

17 Levin, R.P. (2017). Leadership for dentists: It's a good idea to avoid these bad habits. www.dentistryiq.com (accessed 15 December 2018).

18 Ledlow and Coppola (2011). *Leadership for Health Professionals*, 151. Sudbury, MA: Jones and Bartlett Learning.

19 Ledlow and Coppola (2011). *Leadership for Health Professionals*, 171. Sudbury, MA: Jones and Bartlett Learning.

20 Ericsson, K.A., Charness, N., Feltovich, P., and Hoffman, R. (2006). *The Cambridge Handbook of Expertise and Expert Performance*, 440. Cambridge University Press.

21 Ericsson, K.A., Charness, N., Feltovich, P., and Hoffman, R. (2006). *The Cambridge Handbook of Expertise and Expert Performance*, 446. Cambridge University Press.

10

The Office Policy Manual

> *If you don't know where you're going,*
> *you might wind up someplace else.*
> **Yogi Berra**

> *Accepting a leadership position entails having to make difficult choices*
> *and being able to accept that someone else may come up with a better*
> *plan of action. A great leader makes choices based on the association's*
> *best interest, not their own.*
> **John Maxwell**

The Office Policy Manual is not just a "what we do in this office" manual. It is a legal agreement upon which the employer and employee rely on to fulfill each parties' responsibilities to each other. It is a guide, not a contract, for the employee to understand the terms of employment and to resolve employee issues in a mutually agreed-upon manner regarding employment expectations and termination. The Office Policy Manual is perhaps the most important communication that shows leadership to your dental team. Administrative Law Judges, Labor Departments, and the Unemployment Benefits Office often turn to the office manual for guidance in their determinations and rulings for or against the employer. It spells out the terms of employment, including any benefits.

The Office Policy Manual is the main guide for the dentist employer to lead, communicate, and guide employees and when necessary to discipline the employee. It helps when all employees understand the ground rules for employment. It helps form a great team that works together because this becomes the uniform basis for the entire team to follow. It also helps the employer dentist to properly act as the Human Resource Administrator. You, the dentist owner employer, will have to answer employee questions regarding vacation and sick time, cost of dental care for themselves and their families, and use of the phone and computers, to name a few employee issues, along

Leadership and Communication in Dentistry, First Edition. Joseph P. Graskemper.
© 2019 John Wiley & Sons, Inc. Published 2019 by John Wiley & Sons, Inc.

with other benefits, rules, and regulations that the employee may expect, that must be answered by the Human Resource Administrator. If your practice is large enough, you will need an individual to fill this necessary position or outsource these responsibilities to a human resource company.

Due to the many federal and state laws, rules, and regulations that are constantly changing, you should check with a human resource company or employment/labor attorney for direction and advice. A full discussion and legal ramification is beyond the scope of this book. This information is merely a practical guide to gain an understanding of what the Office Policy Manual should cover.

The manual must be written in a clear, decisive, and understandable language so there is no miscommunication. Basic items that should be stated in the Office Policy Manual are that it is not an employment contract, express or implied, and that the manual may be changed with or without notice. Employees will be notified of any changes in a timely manner. The Office Policy Manual must be consistently enforced and applied to all employees. At the beginning you may want to express your office vision statement and mission statement, which is especially helpful to new employees to understand your office "culture." And there should be the statement that this policy supersedes any and all previous written or stated policy. Be sure to review and update on an annual or biennial basis, which should be reissued to each employee and again signed their receipt and understanding of any changes.

Depending on your jurisdiction and the number of employees, workman's compensation, equal opportunity employment, military leave, and family medical leave, to name a few, may have to be written into your Office Policy Manual. If you have over 50 employees, further federal regulations may apply. Therefore, be sure to check with proper legal counsel when writing your office manual such that federal and state requirements, which change with time, are properly fulfilled.

Your mission statement and vision statement should also be placed in the Office Policy Manual so there is no misunderstanding the culture of the practice. It helps that all of staff are focused on the betterment of the practice.

The mission statement is the practice's reason for being. It provides guidance in decision making as well, ensuring that the practice stays on track [1]. The characteristics of a good mission statement should have the following:

1) Mission statements are broadly defined statements of purpose.
2) Mission statements are enduring.
3) Mission statements should underscore the uniqueness of the organization.
4) Mission statements should identify the scope of operations in terms of service and market [2].

True Case (Mission Statement Example) (31)
The entire staff of ABC Dental is committed to providing optimum dental care for all patients in a caring, comfortable, and professional atmosphere where personal attention is given to each and every patient.

The vision statement provides the motivational guidance for the practice and typically defined and promoted by the leadership (you). It provides the practice with a shared image of its direction over the long term. It explains why the organization intends to achieve its goals, whereas mission defines how the practice pursues the goals it does. Together these are called "directional strategies" [1]. The characteristics of a good vision statement should have the following:

1) Describe a practice's organization's big picture and project the future.
2) Be grounded in sound knowledge of the business.
3) Be concrete and as specific as practical.
4) Contrast the present and the future.
5) Stretch the imaginations and creative energies of the people in the practice.
6) Have a sense of significance [3].

True Case (Vision Statement Example) (32)
Our vision is to provide all patients professional care with personal attention that will build a lifelong relationship of trust and confidence to maintain a healthy and happy smile throughout our patient's lives.

At the end of the Office Policy Manual, you should have a signature page acknowledging the employee's receipt and understanding.

Office Hours

First you should make note that the current office hours are always subject to change per the employer. This is to accommodate changes due to patient cancellations, employer vacations, and days off for continuing education. I recommend that staff arrive no more than 15 minutes prior to the patients and all employees must leave as soon as possible after the last patient.

True Case (33)

A dentist with no policy manual noticed that a new employee started to come in 30–40 minutes early before the first patient. When questioned, the employee stated that she came in early to set up the rooms and make sure the computers were on and all was ready to go. The dentist decided to come in an hour early to take note of what was going on. He found that the employee was tending first to her hair and makeup, personal phone calls, and then finally the office duties she claimed doing. This can also happen with an employee staying after to "clean instruments, close down rooms, etc." Both situations gave the employee overtime and allowed other employees to start doing the same or become resentful of the employee getting extra pay.

Time off during office hours and any overtime must have prior approval. If an employee is going to be tardy or absent, they must call in as to the reason. Also, make sure that it is written that continued tardiness and/or absenteeism are grounds for termination.

General Office Rules

General office rules must be stated to clarify the employee's understanding of what is to be expected. State in the Office Policy Manual that all employees are hired "at will" if your jurisdiction allows for it. With an "at-will" employment policy, the employee or the employer may terminate the employment relationship with or without cause and with or without notice. Hence, there is no employment contract or right to employment.

You should also state what you are willing to call full-time and part-time employment. Again, jurisdictions may differ on this issue. If the office is only open 30 hours a week rather than the typical 40 hours, you may want to make an adjustment to the number of hours needed to be considered full-time employment. Later, when benefits are discussed, you are still able to employ the better employee by having benefits available to them even though they are under the traditional 40 hours but still be considered full time. There is a probationary period for all new employees for 90 days, which may be extended if needed and determined by the employer, after which it is not a guarantee of employment nor implicitly promises any additional rights upon completion. Per your jurisdiction, it is a good idea to hire a new possible employee as an independent contractor during the probationary 90 days. This may prevent a new hiree to claim unemployment upon failing during the probationary time. Be sure to have the possible future employee to sign a statement that he or she understands that during the probationary time they will be acting and be paid as an independent contractor and understands all the risks and obligations, including any tax consequences, that are attached to being an independent contractor. It should also be stated that no benefits accrue during this probationary period. Per your jurisdiction a simple statement such as "I hereby understand that I am being hired as an independent contractor. I understand the risks and benefits, including any tax consequences, of being employed as such" may suffice. Again, check with your attorney regarding your jurisdiction.

True Case (34)

After interviewing several applicants for a dental assisting position, the dentist made a choice to have one come in for a working interview. The dentist, only working a half-day over the next couple of days, decided to have the applicant come in the next two half-days. It was an understanding that this was only a working interview and if all goes well he would hire her. Halfway through the second half-day, the dentist informed the applicant of not being hired and was let go. A few weeks later he received a letter that the applicant filed for unemployment on him. He told the unemployment board that she was only there a little more than one half-day for a working interview, not even a full day. He was told that unless indicated otherwise and the applicant was paid for time in the office, he would have to pay unemployment. Hence, the dentist needs to protect the practice by having working interviews sign an agreement/understanding that they will be paid as an independent contractor, if permissible in your jurisdiction.

All employees must adhere to Occupational Safety and Health Administration (OSHA) Bloodborne Pathogen Training and wear the appropriate Personal Protective Equipment (PPE) following proper universal/standard precautions. Gloves, mask, and glasses must be worn whenever involved in patient care. Failure to do so will result in termination. Any and all injuries occurring on the job must be reported immediately to the employer. All required forms must be properly filled out per OSHA Regulations. A note in the policy manual should be made that regulation compliance meetings (covering OSHA, hazard communication, patient emergency protocols, blood-borne pathogen training, waste management, etc.) are regularly held and are mandatory for all.

This office prohibits harassment of any individual based on sex, race, religion, national origin, physical handicap, or age. Any harassment must be reported immediately to the employer in confidence so an investigation may be done and corrective action taken.

Upon termination for any cause, reason, or as determined by the employer, there is absolutely no severance pay to employees.

Social Media

With social media being a very large influential communication tool (both within and outside of the practice), a full understanding by the employee as to the policy and control of usage in regard to the employer and his or her interests must be fully covered. Much damage has been done to employers who have not taken the extra precaution of controlling the social media impact on their practices by employees during their employment and even thereafter if terminated. Social media refers to e-mail, Facebook, Twitter, LinkedIn, Instagram, blogs, and any other electronic communication or activity. Any electronic communication that is found to be defamatory, discriminatory, or offensive in any way regarding the doctor(s), office, practice, and/or fellow employees is completely forbidden and cause for termination. Confidentiality is a must regarding all patient information, and any and all electronic communication must be handled as confidential. The computer and Internet access is for office use, and as such, excessive use of the access to discriminatory, offensive, or obscene sites/uses is ground for termination. The employer reserves the right to monitor all electronic communication including Internet activity in the office.

While employed and after termination all employees and former employees must adhere to Health Insurance Portability and Accountability Act (HIPAA) standards regarding patient information confidentiality and are prohibited from any direct or indirect solicitation of other employees and patients and/or making any disparaging remarks regarding the employer, employees, or patients on or within any electronic communication. This is not intended to regulate employee-to-employee communications but with the intention to protect patient information.

If there is a suspected problem, employee must immediately bring this to the attention of the employer.

During the time of employment and thereafter __Employee's name__ agrees to take no action (written or oral) that is intended or would be reasonably expected to harm __Dentist/employer/dental office__ its/their reputation or that would be reasonably be expected to lead to unwanted or unfavorable publicity to the __Dentist/employer/dental office__.

It is important to spell out how proper interaction, communication, and courtesy to patients should be handled since many people have different personal understandings and cultural basis of what these mean. All employees should have the same way of encountering a patient whether they are new a patient or a patient of many years. All patients should be made to feel special, unique, and respected regardless of how their dental care is paid (cash, PPO insurance, Medicaid, welfare) or how they dress or look. All patients should be greeted by name and a smile to establish identity and feel welcome. When addressing patients younger than mid-twenties, it is permissible to use their first name. However, if the patient is older than the mid-twenties, it is advisable to address them by their last name and the appropriate prefix of Mr., Mrs., Ms., Dr., Fr., Rabbi, Rev., etc. The use of their first name is only allowable with the patient's permission.

In compliance with HIPAA, patients are not to be talked about in front of other people whether in the office or not. Patient confidentiality and patient autonomy must be respected at all times. Any improper and/or discourteous attitudes, communications, or confrontations toward any patient will not be tolerated and will be grounds for termination.

Phone Calls: Office and Personal Cellphones

At times there will be an employee who will use the office phones for excessive personal use. This is not only clogging the incoming calls but also takes away from productive employee time. A policy must be had for employees to understand the total negative impact of excessive personal phone calls on the practice. The office phones are for office business. Personal use of business phones is limited to essential communication or in the case of emergency. Personal phone calls will not be received at work except in an emergency. A message will be taken so you can return the phone call on your own time and not on office time. Excessive office phone or personal employee's cellphone calls (incoming or outgoing) for personal use is cause for termination. Personal cellphones *must* be on silent/airplane mode or off. Employees are prohibited from using cellphone cameras or video recorders on the premise of the practice at any time, and the use of such will result in termination.

Job Duties

There are many job titles within a dental office. Depending on the size of your office, some of your employees will serve several job duties. Below is a list of several job titles most popular within a dental office. Each job title for the jobs you may need, depending on your office size, should have a short list of the major responsibilities of that job. The following are the most common various jobs found in a dental office:

Business Manager
Office Manager
Administrative Assistant
Insurance Coordinator
Financial Coordinator
Communication Coordinator

Appointment Scheduler
Dental Hygienist
Dental Assistant

You can make the list of job duties for each title as short or as long as you wish but make it very clear that the job is not limited to only those items on the list. The list is only to be used as a guide to the employee's responsibilities. Remember with a true team working together and taking individual initiative to go beyond their stated job duties allows the practice to be the best it can be.

My own approach is to have a total cross-trained team where all individuals have some understanding and the capacity to step into any other job. This is especially important in a smaller office. Also in a smaller office, the employees should be able to manage themselves and not have an "office manager," and the dentist employer only gives oversight and direction with proper delegation. This facilitates a more cohesive team for the smaller office.

The following is only an example since each office is different and only intended to be a guide for your own needs:

Front office – Greet patients, attend phones, appointments, insurance processing, recall/maintenance, etc.

Daily

- Open office and turn on all switches in the morning and turn all off at night including computers and monitors.
- Be sure backup system is working daily.
- Set alarm and lock up office.

Weekly

- Water plants.
- Clean counters and front office equipment.
- Organize front reception area including magazines and brochures, as needed.
- Check restroom periodically, as needed, to make sure it is clean.
- Vacuum and clean floors and clean restroom (if you do not have a janitorial service).

Back office – Greet patients, set up and break down operatories, ordering, etc.

Daily

- Clean scrub and sterilize all instruments and handpieces.
- Cold sterile all non-autoclavable items.
- Maintain radiographic images plates.
- Maintain dental supply inventory.

Weekly

- Organize all instrument trays, drawers, and cabinets.
- Vacuum and clean floors in all operatories as needed.
- Test sterilizer with monitor strips.
- Clean/replace, as needed, all suction traps.
- Clean autoclave as needed.

Office Supplies

Stamps, light bulbs, toilet tissue, facial tissues, and dental supplies are all part of the business. Pilferage will be cause for dismissal/termination. This includes pens, pencils, and all other office supplies.

I do mention to the staff that if they need or want something to simply ask. I have always given what was needed. By having them to ask for it even though it is something very small in costs, they are made aware that it is not free and prevents small losses that add up to increased overhead, which you always need to keep under control.

Uniforms

It is always nice to have a dental office team look like a team with the dentist being the leader. It portrays a positive professional office image. You can have anything you want that is appropriate. For examples, some offices like to have each day a different color or always the same color. Due to different styles and fits of clothing, I recommend giving a uniform (scrubs) allowance once a year to allow the employees to purchase their own uniforms within the office guidelines of color and style so all are fitted properly. Therefore, employees are to supply their own uniforms clean and pressed. It should be pointed out that there will be no unprofessional footwear such as flip-flops, sandals, or boots.

Per OSHA, you need to supply and clean PPE for those involved in direct patient care. A PPE allowance should be given to make sure all have proper fitting clinic jackets is easily done when hired.

Personal Grooming

Having hired and fired employees for over 40 years of practice, it always surprised me how great an employee looked at the interview, but after a few months of employment start to look like they slept in their scrubs and haven't taken a shower in days. So it must be noted in the policy manual of what is to be expected in this area.

Hands and fingernails should always be trimmed and clean. Hair should be neat and clean at all times and not interfere with office duties or patient care. Long hair must be pulled back. All makeup application should be done in the restroom and not within patient view and on your own time. Many times the staff would arrive early, clock in, and then apply their makeup. Some would do so in their operatory if a mirror was there. So, after a few incidents, it had to be put into the Office Policy Manual.

All members of the office team should have great oral hygiene after any meal, daily showers, and deodorant. Your employees' appearances help or deter your office image. It is obvious to most employees that proper personal hygiene is necessary in the healthcare office, but I recommend to have it in your Office Policy Manual so all are aware of its importance. There have been situations that were unexpected of an employee continually showing up for work inappropriately.

True Case (35)

After an interview for a new hygienist position, the applicant was hired. At the interview she was professionally dressed. When she showed up for her first day of work, she wore flip-flops, cutoff shorts, and a tee shirt. When asked if she planned to change into something more professional like scrubs, she said, "No. It's a hot day and I always dress casual to put the patient at ease." She was immediately terminated.

Employee Relationships

This is very important to initiate and keep the office upbeat and positive. There is nothing worse than having a "harrumpher" (a person who is a real negative person who harrumphs around the office constantly casting his or her negativity around). Employees are encouraged to cooperate with one another for the good of the practice.

"Teamwork" and helping one another is essential, even if it means going beyond your normal daily duties. Any and all intra-office problems must be immediately brought to the attention of the employer. Bickering and arguing between employees or with the employer when there is a patient in the office, will be grounds for dismissal/termination. Keep communication open and positive at all times.

Discrimination will not be allowed by any employee and should be immediately brought to the attention of the employer and upon investigation may be grounds for dismissal/termination. Dating fellow employees or patients is highly discouraged. If dating does occur with a fellow employee or a patient of record, it must be brought immediately to the attention of the employer.

Staff Meetings

Regardless of the size of your office, you must have regular meetings to keep the team together and on track to build a successful practice. Some offices have daily meetings to keep all of the employees focused on that day's patients. Others only want a weekly or, at the very least, a monthly meeting. It should be stated in the policy manual that meetings are held (daily, weekly, or monthly) or as determined by the employer. Daily meetings are different than monthly meetings in that the daily meeting is to preview the patients appointed that day for full team involvement and completing the schedule in a timely manner. Weekly or monthly meetings are to review any shortcomings or to present new policies, marketing ideas, and improvements in patient care including insurance issues. Staff meetings are mandatory for all employees present that day. It should be pointed out that meetings are for the benefit of all and allows for proper communication to improve patient care. It is *not* a gripe session or used to pick on one employee. I suggest an anonymous suggestion box made available where employees may place suggestions without reprisal. All appropriate suggestions should be covered at the meeting or may be bought to the attention of the employer at any time.

All meetings should be conducted in a very positive manner. There are times when criticism of the team and/or doctor is necessary. To do so, it should be brought up in the middle of the meeting. First open the meeting to involve everyone positively, and then discuss any problems that may be occurring and include the employees to help solve the problem or concern. Approach such a problem or concern as a challenge to solve or how to improve the situation. Leaders learn from the solving of a problem or issue. The dentist leader must lead the team to a solution and not a faultfinding mission. Finish on a positive note summarizing the accomplishments of the meeting and any decisions or recommendations made to make the practice the best it can be.

I have found food as a very good buffer, if needed. I personally have monthly meetings with paid lunch in the office. Most times it is just a short discussion regarding issues of the office to bring the team together. Sometimes problematic issues that affect all must be discussed. When such issues are solved in a positive manner, it brings the team together and unites them. It shows good decisive, can-do leadership.

Employee Breaks

Many jurisdictions have regulations regarding employee breaks. This is normally based on the number of hours you require an employee to work. Be sure to check your jurisdiction's regulations regarding employee breaks. It should be pointed out in your employee policy manual that any break is not to be taken at the expense of the patients' care or if interrupting your front office job duties. All breaks should be taken when and if there is a break between patients. The comfort and care of the patients is of the utmost importance and must be taken into consideration prior to taking any break. The employer, or office manager in a larger office, must be notified of any intended break.

Taking breaks in excessive number or length or if it interferes with patient care is ground for dismissal/termination.

Continuing Education

Again, many jurisdictions have rules and regulations applicable to the employer when requiring employees to attend certain seminars, lectures, or learning events. If you require the employee's attendance, you may have to pay their wages while attending the required course. And always mention that payment for continuing education is at the discretion of the employer, per your jurisdiction. There are times when you see a big benefit for the practice to have the front office personnel attend a seminar that would be specific to the front office. It could also be likewise for the back office. Hence, leaving the decision to pay for the course is at your discretion.

The following must all be true if you do not want to pay the employee:

1) Attendance is outside of normal working hours
2) Attendance is voluntary
3) The employee performs *no* productive work during the event.
4) The seminar is *not* job-related (Fair Labor Standards Act).

You can pay reduced wages for such seminar or training as long as it is not below minimum wage. Exceptions may be granted per your jurisdiction for seminars that are needed to maintain licensure.

Paydays

Paydays must be spelled out as to being weekly, biweekly, twice a month, or whatever you chose. This possibly being your single largest somewhat fixed overhead, be aware of your cash flow to allow a comfortable timing for you the employer.

I highly recommend time card software to maintain fairness to both the employer and the employee. There should not be guesswork in figuring the wages. Estimating an employee's time usually ends in the favor of the employee, especially when they leave a few minutes early for lunch or finish a little earlier than scheduled.

True Case (Example) (36)

If 4 employees arrive just 5 minutes late, leave for lunch 5 minutes early, and leave 5 minutes early at the end of the day, that amounts to 15 minutes paid for 4 employees. That is 60 minutes/day, 300 minutes/week (5 day week), in pay. That doesn't sound like much, but when added up over a period of 1 year (52 weeks), that equals 15 600 minutes (260 hours) per year you are paying! If they are paid $20.00 per hour, you would be paying $5200.60 in unearned wages:

15 minutes × 4 employees = 60 minutes/day
300 minutes/five day week × 52 weeks = 15 600 minutes (260 hours)
260 hours × $20/hour = $5200.00

Time cards are the property of the business. All wages are based on your time card. Any notes regarding mistakes on the time card, sick days, and vacation days must be logged onto your time card accordingly in order to be paid. Any adjustments will be made the next pay period. If payday falls on a holiday, vacation, or when the office is closed, paychecks will be made available before or after accordingly per the employer.

The following items should be included in this section to avoid any miscommunications. No overtime will be paid without prior approval of the employer. Everyone is expected to work as scheduled. Overtime is only paid after 40 hours. (Check with your jurisdiction – it may require overtime to be paid after eight hours.) If you are paying employees based on a salary rather than an hourly wage, other rules do apply. Employees will be evaluated approximately yearly on their anniversary hire date. This is not a guarantee of wage increase or bonus or continued employment. Raises in pay are based on merit only and only at the discretion of the employer. Due to claims of infringement of first amendment rights, you cannot stop employees from talking to each other about their paychecks. You can state that paychecks, wages, bonuses, level of pay, or any other renumeration or gifts are considered to be the employee's confidential information."

To eliminate confusion as to what holidays will be paid or if no holidays will be paid, the policy manual must indicate it. To be paid holiday pay, the employee must have been employed 90 days prior to the holiday. Hence, introductory/probation period and independent contractors are not paid holiday pay, until hired as an employee. If you are going to pay certain holidays, specify which holidays are paid.

I suggest limiting it to only the major ones: New Year's Day, Memorial Day, Independence Day, Labor Day, Thanksgiving Day, and Christmas Day. You can always add another holiday if and when so inclined. When a holiday falls on a vacation day, you will be paid for that day. You will not be paid double for that day (vacation pay and holiday pay) and will not take another day off in place of the holiday. If the holiday occurs during vacation time off, it will be paid as a holiday.

Medical Insurance

Depending on the size and location of your practice, state regulations may have some applicable regulations in this area. So, check with the proper advisor prior to making your decision on whether to include medical insurance benefits or not. Most practices have reduced or eliminated this benefit over the years due to the rapidly rising costs. If you are not going to offer this benefit, state that no medical insurance is offered through the office and may be available to the employee through the State Health Insurance Marketplace. Medical insurance benefits coverage is a fast-changing issue.

The next several sections are about the benefits of the job such as dental care, sick leave, and vacations. Many people take a job based on the hours needed to work, the wages, and the benefits. Although the hours worked and the wages paid to an employee may be specific to the individual employee, dental care, sick time, and vacation time is normally a practice wide benefit. Even if you have a policy regarding employees' personal information, they can still communicate with each other about income and other such benefits. It is very important to maintain a happy and cohesive dental team by keeping all employees included equally based on their length of employment. These policies also become scrutinized by various agencies when unemployment is claimed. Hence, these parts of the manual must be very clear on what is going to be paid and how it is earned.

There will be the employee who will play the benefit game to their advantage, such as to obtain dental care only to leave once it is completed or to work long enough to claim unemployment benefits. This is why I suggest earlier that the possible new employee is hired as an independent contractor with no benefits accruing such that you do not become a victim of such practices.

True Case (37)

A newly hired employee seemed to be a perfect fit for the office. After six months of employment, the employee broke a maxillary anterior tooth and asked if the dentist could fix it. The employee asked if a veneer would be a better restoration than a large composite. Upon examination of the employee, the dentist saw that all for the employee's maxillary anterior teeth were mostly composite restorations that were breaking down due to size. The dentist believed the employee was a good hire and was looking forward to having her as a long-term employee. He proceeded to do six veneers with the understanding that the employee would pay for the lab fees. Once the veneers were in place, the employee never shown up for work again.

Dental Care

Many people seek jobs based on the benefits of having a job in a particular office. Some will seek work in an orthodontic office hoping to get braces, an oral surgeon for implants, or a general dentist for comprehensive dental care for themselves and their families. The employer needs to be fair in providing services to employees so all are treated fairly. You do not want to be the dentist in the above.

True Case (38)
The owner of a large multi-specialty practice had an orthodontist on staff as an associate. The orthodontist would use one of the practice assistants when he was in the office. When the orthodontist decided to leave the practice to set up his own, the assistant left with him. The employee told the owner that if she would go with him, he would do her orthodontics for free. The employee left and two years later, after the orthodontics was completed, asked the previous employer of the multi-specialty practice if she could have her job back since the orthodontics was completed.

No benefits are available prior to 90 days of employment (probationary period). During the first year of employment, all dental benefits are at the discretion of the employer. After one full year of employment, I suggest 50% off regular UCR fees plus any lab fees incurred. You the employer can always do more if so inclined for a certain employee. Routine prophys, X-rays, and exams are at no charge if the employee clocks out. All dental care should be done during slow hours, on the employee's time, and with the employer's knowledge. All appointments should be made with consideration of the scheduling of regular patients. The employee's time card must be properly marked for time taken off for dental care.

If the employee has dental insurance outside of the office, the insurance company will be billed and any payments will be applied to the employee's balance. Spouses and children are given a 50% courtesy off UCR fees plus any lab costs. Other family members should, at your discretion, include the employee's mother and father, brothers, and sisters. They could be given a 20% courtesy off regular UCR fees. No other relatives are included unless you want to expand your inclusion. In the event that the insurance company pays more than 50%, there will not be any refund of the insurance payment to the employee or their families, and it will be applied to the full UCR fee. All insurance forms must be filled out with assignment of payment to the office. Any insurance billing should be billed at the proper adjusted fee so as to not have any false claims being sent.

There are no benefits for part-time employees or independent contractors unless you the employer, at your discretion, want to extend a courtesy.

Any balance due for dental services for employee, spouse, children, or other family member will be taken out of the employee's last paycheck upon termination. This is to protect you from being taken advantage of or providing free/reduced fee dental care and then have the employee leave.

Vacations

Vacation time given as a paid benefit needs to be fully understood and properly communicated to the employee. Normally the vacation time increases as the number of years of employment till a certain level is reached. What is the maximum days of benefit do you the employer want to grant? For example, if giving a total of three weeks off as a benefit after three or five years, it would be good to separate between vacation days and sick days. It is normally more vacation than sick days. So, that would be two weeks' vacation and one-week sick days benefit. Remember that as the employer, especially in a small office, when one employee goes on vacation, either there is lost production or hiring a temporary employee that needs to be paid on top of the vacation benefit being paid. Another reason for cross-training. It is highly suggested that a vacation benefit is only available after the first year of employment and all vacations should be taken when the office is closed. Again, this is especially true for the smaller practice.

All vacation days will be taken prior to any approved personal days, which are without pay. Personal days are days off that may be granted to the employee without pay for various situations. All vacation/personal days must be approved at least two weeks in advance. This allows time to locate a temporary employee if necessary. Paid vacation days are for full-time employees only. There is no paid vacation day benefit for part-time employees. Because employees depend on their pay, vacation days may be used when the office is closed due to inclement weather or any other reason; otherwise the employee is not paid when the office is closed.

Vacations days should not be carried over to the next year and will be lost/forfeited if not used by the employee's anniversary hire date. It must be spelled out that there is no accrual for vacation days, if this is allowable by your jurisdiction. If so, state that vacation days are merely a gratuitous courtesy and not an accrued benefit.

For ease of calculations, vacation benefit days should be broken down to half-days to allow the employee to take a half a day when necessary. With our example, the first week of vacation would be granted after one year of employment and be taken during the second year of employment as it applies to their anniversary hire date. During the third year of employment, another week may be granted (I normally make this the one week of sick leave). If you are a small office, it can be noted that the two weeks may not be taken consecutively due to the impact on the office.

By the end of the third year of employment, another week is added to the vacation if you so desire, which gives the employee three weeks of paid (vacation and sick) leave days. You can offer more or less depending on your ability to provide the benefits offered.

Usually there are not many problems of days owed with long-term employees. It is when they are terminated or quit during the first couple of years. So you need a policy to cover those situations of when the employee, whether short term or long term, leave the practice for whatever reason.

If employment is terminated during the first year of employment, any and all vacations days are forfeited. Again, check your jurisdiction that such forfeiture is allowed. If employment is terminated after the first year of employment, all vacations days are forfeited, and a possible courtesy in consideration for the time employed may be granted at the discretion of the employer.

If employment is terminated on good terms with the employer and allowing a two-week notice to the employer of the employee's termination, as a courtesy to the employee and after forfeiture of all vacation days, there may be a pro-rated payment of 0.134 day per full week worked during the current employment year from the anniversary employment date to the date of termination and is determined by the cause for termination and at the discretion of the employer.

Sick Leave

You can have a very strict policy requiring a doctor's note to confirm that the employee was actually sick or you can have a very loose policy with no requirements and allowing sick leave to be taken for any personal reason. When an employee calls in sick unexpectedly, you as the leader of the office team need to either delegate the responsibility to another employee to make sure the position is covered or arrange the appointment schedule to accommodate one less staff member. Either way creates an impact on the office production. Therefore, it is wise to have a policy that encourages the employee not to take sick days unless absolutely sick enough not to come in. So after a period of time (after the second year of employment in the example above), once sick days are granted as a benefit, unused sick days are paid at $50.00 per day. This is paid on top of the earned wages. This rewards the employee and keeps the office production up without interference of employees not being at work. Again sick days are a gratuitous courtesy and not an accrued benefit.

To continue with our example from the vacation days, after two years' employment, full-time employees will be eligible for one-week paid sick leave (as broken down by half-days worked, if you want). If and when sick, the employer must be notified before the start of work on the day you are missing due to sickness. Failure to do so is cause for dismissal/termination. Sick days are only used if you are too sick to come to work. Under a strict policy using sick days for any other reason is cause for dismissal/termination and will not be paid. Under a looser policy, sick days may be taken as personal days without any given reason. Sick leave is not accrued and cannot be accumulated. The maximum sick days allowed in one anniversary period is one week. Depending on your how strict you want to be, if more than two sick days in a row, a doctor's verification is necessary to receive sick leave pay. There is no sick leave before two years' employment. Upon termination, with or without cause, all sick days are forfeited.

It should be pointed out that the area of vacation, sick, and personal days is a constantly changing area of labor law and as such proper legal advice is advised.

True Case (39)

An employee of eight years was fired. When she applied for unemployment benefits, requesting vacation days and sick days, the dentist appealed the granting of benefits to the former employee. He included a copy of the Office Policy Manual that stated if an employee was terminated with cause, the employee loses all vacation and sick days. After the appeal, a date was set for the dentist and the former employee to meet with an Administrative Law Judge. The former employee showed up with an attorney. The decision was made for the former employee based on the wording of the Office Policy Manual that did use the word "loses," but not have the word "forfeit," which the Administrative Law Judge decided was a better word and should have been used.

Other Benefits

There are many other benefits that you can grant to your employees. Some jurisdictions and depending on the number of employees, there may applicable federal and state rules and regulations that dictate certain benefits that must be granted to the employees. Other benefits could include:

Bonuses based on office production/collection or individual goals
Pension plan

Continuing education
Life insurance
Maternity leave
Military leave
Day care

Always keep in mind that once a benefit is granted, it is very hard to take it away when the economy or office income shrinks. Hence, good leadership keeps the bigger long-term view of the practice and how to properly manage the employees for the benefit of the practice, the employees, and yourself.

Confidentiality and Acknowledgment

(This last section must be signed by the employee and you must keep a copy of their signature agreeing with this policy.)

As was mentioned before, you need to protect the practice from employees taking information from the practice or giving practice information to anyone outside of the practice.

All employees agree that any and all patient charts, files, and lists shall belong to and are the sole and exclusive property of the practice and the employer. All employees further agree and acknowledge that the patient charts, files, and lists and the information contained therein and the names and addresses of all patients are confidential and constitute trade secrets of the employer. All employees further promise and agree that he or she will not disclose such confidential information including office policy and office management information and procedures to any other person or electronic/social media and shall not use such confidential information other than in connection with their employment with the practice. The intent of this policy is not to regulate employee to employee communications but to protect patient information.

This policy may be reviewed by the employer and changes may be made without notice based on the sole discretion of the employer and the employee to be informed in a timely manner. No statement of policy as set forth in this policy manual is intended as a contractual commitment or obligation of the employer of the office or any other individual employee or group of employees. Circumstances may arise in which the employer determines that changes in these policies are required. For this reason, the employer reserves the right, at any time, to modify, rescind, or supplement any and all action that may be contrary to a policy set forth herein with notice to the employees.

During the time of employment and thereafter __Employee's name__ agrees to take no action (written or oral) that is intended or would be reasonably expected to harm __Dentist/employer/dental office__ its/their reputation or that would be reasonably be expected to lead to unwanted or unfavorable publicity to the __Dentist/employer/dental office__.

I have read, understand, and agree to this office policy.

_____

Employee Signature   Date

References

1 Ledlow, G.R. and Coppola, M.N. (2011). *Leadership for Health Professionals*, 142. Sudbury, MA: Jones and Bartlett Learning.
2 Swayne, L.E., Duncan, W.J., and Ginter, P.M. (2006). *Strategic Management of Health Care Organizations*, 5e, 191–192. Malden, MA: Blackwell, note 2.
3 Lerner, H. (2003). Visions Statements. *Beyond Numbers*, p. 9.

Section 3

Leadership, Communications, and Success for Your Self

Leadership begins with the leader discovering and incorporating leadership qualities in themselves to make their self to be the best you, you can be. With true leadership of self you will be able to balance your life to live life successfully.

Leadership and Communication in Dentistry, First Edition. Joseph P. Graskemper.
© 2019 John Wiley & Sons, Inc. Published 2019 by John Wiley & Sons, Inc.

11

Understanding Leadership

The quality of a leader is reflected in the standards they set for themselves.
Ray Kroc

The only man who never makes a mistake is the man who never does anything.
Theodore Roosevelt

Discussions of leadership have been had almost from the beginning of time. There has always been the question: "Who is going to be the leader?" In answering that question, a consensus usually responds by choosing that person with certain qualities that the majority feel safe and secure to follow. The basis for their selection may be based on looks, intelligence, inherited bloodlines, or what may be offered by the selected leader. That majority may select and follow the leader, whether good, bad, or even evil, to promote their needs, wants, desires, and beliefs. This does not pertain to dictatorships, military juntas, or other non-majority selected leaders who obtained leadership by force. However, it is the leader's attributes that bring the majority together for the leader's support. Without support from the majority, leadership is lost. This is also true for the successful dental office.

With all the stakeholders involved in the success of your practice, there are also many others that influence the leader in his or her decision making. There are fellow colleagues, supply vendors, social media, dental labs, dental equipment and computer repair personnel, landlord, and accountant, to name just a few. These are considered outside influencers. Inside influencers are the staff, patients, family, marketing, management systems, conflict resolution, and many more. You must know your self as to how much influence to allow others to have over you. You must know your employees as to how much change they will allow to advance the practice and what are you going to do with those who do not.

There are many theories on what makes up a leader. The concept and discussion of leadership is ancient; the discipline of leadership study can be consistently traced back to Machiavelli in 1530, with the first documentation of leadership dating back to 2300 BC [1]. As early as 400 BC, Greek philosopher Xenophon first described leadership based on traits of leaders of his time, which were based on military leadership. Courage and mastery of horsemanship were valuable leadership tools, along with heritage. The first theories that were popular from approximately 450 BC to the 1940s were the "Great Man" (also Great Woman such as Joan of Arc) Theory and the Trait Theory. Under these theories, studies were done to determine what specific traits make a person an effective leader [2]. In 1530, Machiavelli promoted his Narcissist Theory that good leaders should be malevolent and feared. Fear should be used as a motivator [3]. Hence, he promoted the theory that "The end justifies the means." This theory lasted till about 1840 when the Great Man Theory was promoted by the researchers Carlyle, Galton, and James [4]. They studied the traits of great men and found that many leaders had immutable traits such as gender, race, height, and oration and mutable traits such as social class, education, and religion [4]. This progressed till the 1940s.

In the 1940s till the 1960s, the Behavioral Theory began to develop, which had two parts: Theory X and Theory Y [5]. Theory X relied on the behavior of a non-leader being not motivated, disliked work, no self-discipline, and no responsibility. I call this group non-achievers. Applying this to the dental practice, the dentist's leadership style is one of complacency and is content with mediocrity. This type of dentist leader is happy just to maintain the status quo. They allow the practice to run unimproved, without true leadership involvement, and give no direction or team motivation for practice improvement. Theory Y, on the other hand, viewed the behavior of a leader as motivated, liked to work, had self-discipline, and took on responsibility. This dentist's leadership style is one of motivation to achieve the best available outcome from the endeavors of all in the practice – patients, staff, and self. This type of dentist leader views problems as challenges and is pragmatic and innovative with a "can-do" attitude.

There are several types of leadership style in use. To discuss all would be beyond the scope of this book; hence I shortly discuss those most applicable: Organizational, Transformational, Omnibus, Situational/Contingency, and Dynamic Culture.

Organizational leaders lead through managerial skills. They tend to take more of a back seat to a leadership role. They like to maintain the status quo because the practice is "running like a well-oiled machine." Don't rock the boat. Here the practice will not grow and eventually will not be able to sustain itself and ultimately fail.

Transformational leaders lead through their ability to connect with others being the patients, staff, and vendors. They tend to have charisma giving them very strong emotional appeal and good visionary communication that inspires and stimulates subordinates/staff. Here the practice will grow by motivating the staff and patients by providing clear visionary goals.

Omnibus leaders lead through a more traditional focus on the various outcomes to describe who they are and how they lead. More emphasis is given to the results of his or her leadership outcomes to give meaning. Here a practice becomes dependent on the leader to provide success. The practice will grow but never reach its full potential without being a team.

Situational/contingency leaders lead through the situation given. There is no one way to lead. They tend to be most adaptable to use the proper leadership skill applicable to the situation. The practice will do very well with this type of leadership but may need some goal setting to reach its true potential.

Dynamic culture leaders optimize the leadership potential as much as possible knowing it is not possible at all times in a dynamic setting of diversity, Internet, and technology in today's world. The practice will be successful and flourish because there is a continuity to strive to be the best it can be.

Superb leadership now is required at all levels due to the dynamic and cultural influences on the leader. Hence the Dynamic Cultural Leadership (DCL) Model is most applicable to the dentist leader. The Dynamic Cultural Leader understands the following needs and influences:

Increased diversity in thinking and allow to be open to new ideas
Increased access to information to the point of overload for the dentist, staff, and the patients
Increased patient sophistication
Increased speed of the Internet
Increased evolution of technology

All of this is influencing the culture embedded in the practice shareholders (dentist, staff, and patients) and in that which the dentist leader intends to instill in the organization/practice. Culture is a learned system of knowledge, behavior, attitudes, beliefs, values, and norms that are shared by a group of people [6].

The leadership model you choose will be based on your personal values and experiences. Leading ethically is also a key in your leadership style. Your interaction with others in the way you treat other people and your willingness to turn mistakes into learning experiences and humility will guide you in developing your leadership style. You will incorporate the right leadership model, framework, or combination of skills and techniques into your personal and professional life with the best choices to allow you to be the best you, you can be.

You must be open-minded and able to adapt as the unknown becomes known. As Donald Rumsfeld stated regarding a leader's knowledge, "There are known knowns: things we know we know. There are known unknowns: things that we know we don't know. But there are also unknown unknowns – things we do not know we don't know." Being conscious of these three caveats allows the dentist leader to appreciate the challenges of leadership in understanding and the knowledge needed in the dynamic culture in which he or she must lead.

There are three levels that a leader must include in his or her recipe for success: organizational level (your patients/practice), team level (your staff), and personal level (your self) [7]. All three must be listened to, understood, and included in the leader's decision making.

The study of leadership began to look at the technical skills, human skills, conceptual skills, and administrative skills that a leader would need to be successful. The competent leader must have these skills that make the leader accountable. Technical skills are those skills that require knowledge and ability. The dentist leader needs to not only know technical, specialized skills but must also continue a lifelong quest to always improve and build upon that knowledge and skill. He or she also needs to continually train and upgrade their staff's knowledge and skills to have continued enhancement of the practice. The dentist leader must have the ability to see what knowledge and skills are necessary to seek out for continued success. Merely taking continuing education courses or buying expensive equipment that are not relevant or able to be incorporated into the practice is not good leadership. It would be a waste of time, money, and effort if never used or implemented. Therefore, the dentist leader must have creativity, innovation, risk-taking, and the ability to give some direction in bringing new ideas that are worthy of exploration for the team to excel. The knowledge or skill sought by the dentist or staff must be applicable and able to be incorporated into the practice to be considered a good leadership decision.

Human or interpersonal skills are those skills that require knowledge of interpersonal relationships, understanding human behavior, and having a good perception of other's motivation, needs, and wants to build upon, thereby creating an effective leadership/follower relationship. The dentist leader must understand not just his staff's but also his or her patients' motivation, needs, and wants. Having this skill set allows the dentist to lead the practice, patients and staff, to achieve success for all, avoid adverse outcomes, and intercede and/or eliminate any conflicts that occur. The biggest component in interpersonal relationships is communication: not just what is said but how it is said. This includes the leader's understanding of the emotional maturity, personal attitude, and motivations of those he or she leads.

Conceptual skills are those skills that require analytical and logical thinking to create and develop ideas that can be useful to those being lead. The dentist leader must be able to break down complex situations and problems to be easily identified and dealt with by patients and staff. The leader must fully engage the culture in which he or she wants their practice to operate. If the dentist leader does not create, communicate, and fully engage the basis upon which the practice stands for, no one else will. Mastering conceptual skills allows the dentist leader to become transformational and not just a reactionary leader.

Administration skills are those skills that require understanding and the ability to perform all necessary managerial functions. The dentist leader must be able to do the day-to-day jobs of hiring, firing, budgeting, supply management, coaching and rules/regulation compliance, and staff meetings. Many of these skills may be delegated to an office manager or even a dental management organization (DMO)/dental support organization (DSO). However, the more that is delegated, the more the practice will take on that other's belief of what the practice culture should be and not that of the dentist owner. This is especially true for the smaller practice where there are fewer staff members and one staff member has been delegated the role of "office manager." Without oversight by the owner dentist, the practice culture will revert to the office manager's idea of what the dental practice should be and place his or her ideas and beliefs on the forefront of the practice goals. This can happen unintentionally as more is delegated to a non-owner leader. If what was delegated is basically the control of the practice and the owner dentist is merely the producer of services, who does not want to take a managerial role in the practice, the practice leadership defers to the office manager. This is not the same as a large office or a practice with multiple locations delegating managerial duties to certain individuals at the individual practice location. Leadership duties should still be retained by the owner. It is in the allowing of an office manager to take only a limited role in the leadership of the office/practice that allows the dentist leader to retain true leadership with proper delegation of duties.

Are you going to just manage your practice or are you going to lead your practice? It is important to understand the differences of a being a manager and a leader of your practice. It is possible to be both, as are most owner dentists. Managers are mission oriented with shorter time/vision viewpoint. A good manager has excellent reliable organizational skills allowing for improved staff performance. Most managers have a good skill set that enables the management of all the practice resources. Leadership is more than just skills. Leaders have a longer time/vision viewpoint. A good leader envisions and develops long-term goals that enables and maintains practice growth. There has been much literature on the dentist owner being the CEO of his or her practice. For a successful practice, the owner dentist must be more than just a CEO. There are many corporations that have CEOs that have misled the corporation into insolvency. Hence, not all CEOs are leaders. To be a successful CEO, you must be a dentist with great leadership skills.

Managers manage resources, while leaders lead people. Hence, it is important to hire individuals that are able to manage themselves especially in a smaller office. This is most important in developing a highly motivated staff. When employees are able to manage themselves, they take more initiative and have more enjoyment in fulfilling their job duties because they will have a sense of importance and inclusion. They will become motivated with this newfound empowerment. This new empowerment of the employee allows the dentist leader to give more time and effort to leadership and not just manage the practice. Of course, there will be a certain staff member that rises to the level to become the one person the owner dentist goes to help run the practice. However, when that takes place, it is important for the owner dentist to ensure that true management powers are not handed over to that staff member unless it is so intended. Keeping all staff members completely accountable to manage their performance is very important to building a true team. There will be those that do not measure up to this newfound empowerment. Management guru Peter Drucker said, "Management is doing things right; leadership is doing the right things."

One of the main attributes of a leader is competency. It has been found that there are basically four levels of competency, much like Donald Rumsfeld's three caveats:

1) Unconscious incompetence – "We do not know what we do not know."
2) Conscious incompetence – "We know that we do not know."
3) Conscious competence – "We know how to perform a skill but must consciously think about it."
4) Unconscious competence – "We perform the skill as second nature" [8].

Level 1 – Remember year 1 of dental school? Without a mentor or a person to guide an individual, the person will be stuck at level 1 until an event or a situation occurs to force the person to rise to level 2. This is the dentist who does not rise above graduation from dental school. He or she does not make any effort to improve their skills until something goes wrong for a patient or the practice. They are then motivated to level 2 to correct the situation.

Level 2 – This is much like year 2 of dental school. A good leader will seek a mentor or other professional respective to the situation to guide them or learn from them to allow level 3 to be obtainable. At this level the dentist will seek out numerous postgraduate education courses and/or mentors to improve and build his or her knowledge and skills.

Level 3 – Year 3 struggles to perform a procedure should come to mind. A good leader will practice, fine-tune, and hone the learned leadership skills so they will rise to level 4. Not only does this dentist take the courses but actually brings that knowledge back to the practice and applies it in the effort to continually improve the care and skills learned at level 2.

Level 4 – Year 4 and residency brings you to a higher level of performance. At this level the leader has a skill set that has become so ingrained in the person that it becomes automatic normal behavior for the leader to build upon. It becomes part of the leader's "DNA." At this level the dentist now has accomplished complete application of the knowledge or skills learned such that there is little thought in their application.

Most successful leaders fully understand the importance of each competency level and its impact on their decisions and leadership growth. To achieve the highest level of competence, one must practice the skill, trait, or management style often, with proper direction, feedback, and a continuous yearning to learn what works and was does not. Successful leaders have discipline, persistence, and humility while continuously working to improve their capabilities.

Dye and Garmen cite 16 competencies for healthcare executives, which includes the owner dentist regardless of number of staff or size of office, that are based on 4 cornerstones of exceptional leadership:

Cornerstone 1 (A): Well-cultivated self-awareness
Cornerstone 2 (B): Compelling vision
Cornerstone 3 (C): Real way with people
Cornerstone 4 (D): Masterful style of execution [9]

A) A well-cultivated self-awareness (Know thy self!)

1) Living by personal convictions (Live what you believe)
2) Possessing emotional intelligence (Must be self-reflective)
   It is perhaps one of the most important competencies for a leader to know who they are through self-reflection and actually living what they believe. Not just talk the talk but to also walk the walk. Say what you mean and mean what you say. To enhance personal convictions, one must have daily affirmations that guide the leader's mindset to fulfill his or her goals.

   These competencies lead to the consistency of behavior and temperament and having the emotional intelligence to allow one to have the ability to monitor self and social settings, thereby allowing one to govern behavior accordingly.

B) Compelling vision (Must have a goal to achieve)

3) Being visionary (Must be able to create the visionary dream goal)
4) Communicating vision (Must be able to convincingly describe the goal)
5) Earning loyalty and trust (Being truthful, sincere, and trustworthy – Keeping your word)
   Every true leader has a clear vision of their goals and a plan to achieve them. It should be pointed out that long-term planning is not the same as a compelling vision. No one starts or buys a dental practice without having a goal, a vision, or a dream of what they want to achieve. A dream written down with a date becomes a goal. A goal broken down into steps becomes a plan. A plan backed by action makes your dreams come true [10]. A dentist leader not only has a goal but also a plan to establish a practice or enhance and elevate a bought practice. He or she knows

they cannot achieve the goal of a successful practice without others (a dedicated and motivated staff). Communication of the goal and the plan is paramount so the staff can also visualize it and "buy into it." Without staff-followers, the dentist leader is alone in his or her pursuit and unable to fulfill his or her set goals.

To develop a goal-oriented team practice, you must have an office culture that all of the staff team take hold and believe. The office culture can be based on your mission statement and your vision statement as discussed in Chapter 10. But it takes more than just statements to build a successful professional life and practice. It takes a culture or belief that brands a practice. Branding a practice is more than a logo, symbol, or jingle. It represents the unique value of the practice and how the entire staff, including the dentist, interacts with the public and more importantly the patients. It is the sum of all promises and perceptions a practice wants its patient base and the supporting community to believe about the practice's products and services. Patients and the community the practice is located in will attach a psychological meaning and value to your practice based on the culture you exhibit in your practice and beyond when active in the community. To be successful, the perceived value the patient places on the services you provide must be greater than or equal to the price paid. Therefore, patients must believe that the services they received were well worth the price paid.

There are various ways patients place value on your services. It could be because you offer and help with their dental insurance, accept payment plans, and have a friendly staff, or simply because you give painless injections.

The staff must buy in and fully believe in the office culture and the branding. This is shown to patients by exemplifying the culture/brand in their interactions with the patients at all times. Of course, the dentist leader must "talk the talk and walk the walk" to lead the staff in his or her efforts to build a successful practice. You must live, eat, and breathe the practice brand/culture because if you do not, who will? Personal discipline to work a little longer and a little hard without strain engenders respect while it educates and acclimates lower staff members. This can be accomplished by bonding with employees for culture brand, respecting employees as people, and modeling the attitude they should have toward patients.

To give incorrect or improper communication or not keeping your word with the staff would be a sure way to never achieving your goals. The staff will always pick up on an untrustworthy leader "wannabe" when their word has not been kept, follow-through is absent, and constant communication with the staff is missing. They will not follow and the practice will stagnate or even fail.

These competencies lead to communication, knowledge, skills, and abilities that need to be in place, which means that the leader knows how, what, and when to communicate important information and how to become known as authentic and genuine.

C) Real way with people (Understanding of others)

6) Listening like you mean it (Focus on what someone is saying and not on what you want to say)
7) Giving back (Be a giver, not a taker)
8) Mentoring others (Openly being helpful and honest to those that ask)
9) Developing teams (Understand others' strengths and weaknesses)
10) Energizing staff (Must be the biggest cheerleader of the team by enabling the strengths and building up the weaknesses)

Great leaders are true team players who actually and fully become a team member and not just one who gives orders. By listening and giving back to the team individually and collectively, you will enable the development of the team's culture. Listening is more than just hearing. Listening is active while hearing is passive.

When listening to a staff member or patient, you actually take part by acknowledging what they are saying by paraphrasing back to the person what you received and understood to show your understanding of what they said. Also asking questions engages both parties. It shows active listening and concern for what is being said. By active listening, trust will be earned. Each member, as well as the team, needs to be understood so the team building can be productive.

It is also very important to show you are one of the team especially in a smaller office where there are only one to three doctors. This is easily shown by simply doing any of the menial tasks of maintaining the office, from picking things off the floor or taking out the trash to cleaning an operatory if an assistant is a little behind or making an appointment for a patient when others are already busy. There are many small tasks you can do to show your involvement as a fellow team member. In other words, do not ask someone to do something that you are not willing to do your self.

Developing a team to reach its full potential also requires a lot of cheerleading for the things that go right and to boost up morale when things are not so right. Congratulate the success and encouragement to do better when needed. Positive rewards including a single "Thank you" or a "Job well done" do not go unappreciated, but also bring about positive reactions and continued growth.

These competencies will give the leader understanding of the powerful relationship of trust and understanding. Increased trust leads to greater understanding, and increased understanding in turn leads to greater trust, hence allowing true team building to exist.

D) Masterful execution (Must have discipline and persistence)

11) Generating informal power (Maintaining a knowledge base and caring attitude that allows staff to reach their potential because they know they are helpful not because the boss made me do it)

12) Building consensus (Listen to all and have all feel they are heard and considered)

13) Making decisions (Making the decision that will be best for all)

14) Driving results (Must make all accountable for the success)

15) Stimulating creativity (Pay attention to new ideas that may surface)

16) Cultivating adaptability (Not every decision is successful but how one adapts and learns is essential) [11].

Leaders are consistent in their staff's development. They also hold the line on allowing mediocrity to set in individually or within the team as a whole. Therefore, discipline is very important for the doctor and the staff to know the acceptable limits and boundaries of the office culture. Along with discipline comes adaptability from which the doctor must listen to the staff when there needs to be a change in the office culture or in the leader themselves to accommodate changes in the patients' needs or changes in the insurance/business structure under which the office works.

These competencies lead to:

Integrity that makes communication fair and balanced

Integrity in both on and off the job

Integrity in self-monitoring to act morally and ethically

Integrity in putting other's (person or organization) interest before and above their own

So what is the definition of leadership? I have found the definition of Ledlow and Coppola to be on target. Leadership is the dynamic and active creation and maintenance of an organizational culture and strategic systems that focus the collective energy of both leading people and managing resources toward meeting the needs of the external environment utilizing the most efficient, effective, and efficacious methods possible by moral (ethical and legal) means [11].

Ledlow and Coppola further describe leader success:

$$\text{Leader Success} = \text{Individual (Nature} + \text{Nurture)} \times \text{Situational} \\ \text{Adaptation} \times \text{Organization Culture Creation} \times \\ \text{Personal} + \text{SubordinateAccountability [12].}$$

For the dentist leader, leadership success is you (who you are plus what you have learned in life) multiplied by how you can properly adapt and react to various situations that may occur, multiplied by the practice vision and culture you have created, multiplied by your own accountability for the direction your practice is going, plus holding your staff accountable for the duties given to them to fulfill the mission and vision of the practice. However, is that the real definition of being successful at living? As will be pointed out, there is more to success than just a successful practice.

Owner dentists must establish the office culture by which the staff and patients buy into. He or she must focus the entire energy of the practice (staff and resources) to the success of patient care (physically, financially, and emotionally), which in turn provides the very best practice. He or she must also keep up to date and adaptable to the ever-changing improvements in patient care and staff management.

Are these competencies a born trait or can they be learned and exercised? It is both. Many leaders have been self-taught but also have an inner belief in themselves to be leaders. There are also those who by nature of their placement in society are automatically given a leadership position. However, being given a leadership position is only part of the equation – they must measure up to the expectation of being a leader or they will not succeed. Therefore, there is a learning element to being a leader. Great leaders are always on the move to learn more about themselves, their business, the world, and the people around them. There is no "one" way to lead. You must grow into your own leadership style by constantly learning and trying various leadership styles. You will eventually default to the style of leadership that is comfortable and beneficial to you and those around you such that you will become successful at living. You will achieve level 4 of leadership competency.

References

1 Ledlow, G.R. and Coppola, M.N. (2011). *Leadership for Health Professionals*, 57. Sudbury, MA: Jones and Bartlett Learning.
2 Ledlow, G.R. and Coppola, M.N. (2011). *Leadership for Health Professionals*, 58. Sudbury, MA: Jones and Bartlett Learning.
3 Ledlow, G.R. and Coppola, M.N. (2011). *Leadership for Health Professionals*, 60. Sudbury, MA: Jones and Bartlett Learning.
4 Ledlow, G.R. and Coppola, M.N. (2011). *Leadership for Health Professionals*, 61. Sudbury, MA: Jones and Bartlett Learning.
5 Ledlow, G.R. and Coppola, M.N. (2011). *Leadership for Health Professionals*, 63. Sudbury, MA: Jones and Bartlett Learning.
6 Schein, E.H. (1999). *The Corporate Culture Survival Guide: Sense and Nonsense About Culture Change*. San Francisco, CA: Jossey-Bass Note 99.

7 Schein, E.H. (1999). *The Corporate Culture Survival Guide: Sense and Nonsense About Culture Change*, 191. San Francisco, CA: Jossey-Bass.

8 Schein, E.H. (1999). *The Corporate Culture Survival Guide: Sense and Nonsense About Culture Change*, 7. San Francisco, CA: Jossey-Bass.

9 Dye, C.F. and Garman, A.N. (2006). *Exceptional Leadership*, xxi. Chicago, IL: Health Administration Press.

10 http://www.azquotes.com/author/49648-Greg_Reid (accessed 24 June 2018).

11 Ledlow, G.R. and Coppola, M.N. (2011). *Leadership for Health Professionals*, 15. Sudbury, MA: Jones and Bartlett Learning.

12 Ledlow, G.R. and Coppola, M.N. (2011). *Leadership for Health Professionals*, 85. Sudbury, MA: Jones and Bartlett Learning.

12

Your Self

There is only one corner of the universe you can be certain of improving, and that is your own self.
Aldous Huxley

What we think, we become.
Buddha

Excellence is an art won by training and habituation. We do not act rightly because we have virtue or excellence, but rather have those because we have acted rightly. We are what we repeatedly do. Excellence, then, is not an act but a habit.
Aristotle

Leadership and communication with your practice and your patients are an extension of you and will only be true as you are to your self to become the best you, you can be. All great leaders, whether good or bad, have a great understanding of who they are, where they want to go, and what they have to do to get there. We have already discussed the concepts of born leaders and self-made leaders in Chapter 11. But how do you get knowledge of your self such that it defeats outside influences not conducive to you or your goals?

Leadership of self is tied to self-communication that results in living successfully. In order to lead one's self, you must know and understand who you are. You must have knowledge of self. As mentioned in Chapter 11, Aristotle's "Know thy self" is perhaps the most important attribute in living life success-fully. A true self-reflection entails honestly evaluating your positives and your negatives that create the composite person you are. This is absolutely imperative to becoming the best you, you can be. It is a lifelong journey with an effort to be successful through continuing education for the patient, seeking proper

Leadership and Communication in Dentistry, First Edition. Joseph P. Graskemper.
© 2019 John Wiley & Sons, Inc. Published 2019 by John Wiley & Sons, Inc.

business advice for the practice, and proper self-reflection and improvement for your self to become the best version of you.

There are many codes of ethics that many dentists turn to guide them in their practice. However, they are not a guide to successful living. They are guides to proper ethical professional behavior. You also need to have a code for your self. To do this you must not only know thyself, but you must have knowledge of your self.

Many dentists want to only be a manager of their practice and not truly lead the practice to the next level. This is equally important in the pursuit of living life successfully. Not every dentist wants or should be the leading force of the practice. But to know which you are is paramount in becoming the best you, you can be. To do so, you must understand your self. The acceptance and realization of your personal view of what success is will lead you to living successfully or being successful at living. Being a single provider practice or a multi-location multi-specialty practice requires the leader or manager dentist in both situations to know thy self.

To get to that level of self-reflection, you need to understand the importance of the brain versus mind. The brain is anatomical, while the mind is the mechanism that exhibits the results of the brain working, such as "What's on your mind?" There have been shown that there are different levels of the brain functioning: Beta, Alpha, Theta, and Delta. Each level represents a deeper level of consciousness from awake, subconscious, and unconscious [1]. Many thoughts in the subconscious guide your leadership decision making. They occur as the proverbial "light bulb" that goes off when you are in a quiet state, as found in sleep, deep thought, or during a mindful quiet time. A complete discussion is beyond the scope of this book, but some basics are needed to understand the necessary steps to discovering the best you, you can be.

Many ask: where do I start to learn how to self-reflect? First, after an understanding of the following concepts as they apply to you personally, you must go to a "quiet spot." Some may call it meditation, while others will call it a small time-out to reassess what is happening in your life. Whatever you want to call it, you need a little "quiet time," which means really quiet – no input. The best most can achieve in reality is driving without the radio on, sitting quietly somewhere (beach/park/porch or patio), or time spent on a treadmill. It is merely time to take for your self. Mindfully close your eyes (if possible) and visualize where you want to be in your personal and professional life 5, 10, and 20 years from this current point. Live that visualization and keep it alive as your goal that is totally obtainable. Act as if you already have obtained the visualization to make an affirmation of what is to become. A visualization of a goal must occur prior it any manifestation of that goal. Of course, over time one's life and goals will change, and therefore the 5-, 10-, and 20-year visualization will change to accommodate your want to be successful at living.

To start an exercise in self-reflection, mentioned before, you must know and understand your self, regarding these areas:

1) Your personality.
2) Your learning style.
3) Your style of leadership.
4) Your skills and weaknesses.
5) Your natural abilities (creativeness vs. details).
6) Your moral compass [2].

Your personality and manner of learning, which leads to your style of leadership, with an understanding of your skills and weaknesses, as they relate to your natural abilities, led by a moral compass, can be broken down in several ways: emotional intelligence, hemisphere dominance, Jungian assessment, A-B indicators, Visual, Aural, Read/write, and Kinesthetic sensory modalities (VARK) Test, and New Enneagram Test [3].

Emotional intelligence has four constructs: self-awareness, self-management, social awareness, and social skills [4]. These are needed in being a dynamic cultural leader, as pointed out in Chapter 11, to have the ability to apply art and science introvertantly and extrovertantly:

1) Self-awareness is understanding one's personal strengths and weaknesses and, more importantly, how these affect others. This fosters an ability to accept creative criticism and actually learn from it.
2) Self-management is the ability to express emotions without complete abandon. There is a maturity evident in the dispersal of feelings delivered with restraint. This also goes to one's motivation that strongly defends against disappointment and obstacles, an unflagging optimism fueling an inner ambition.
   In other words, good leader have big egos. Great leaders know how to control it.
3) Social awareness is the ability to build rapport and a sense of community within your practice and to instill trust within a group. Power struggles and ego clashes are overridden by a genuine appreciation for what others bring to the table.
4) Social skills are your interactions with patients and staff within your practice, fellow colleagues, and those in your community using an understanding of human nature coupled with the spirit of compassion. Showing empathy within your social skills allows for a deeper personal connection and generates direct response to another's adversity.

Hemisphere dominance relates to which side of the brain we use more in our daily activities. Right-sided persons tend to be more creative and entrepreneurial, while left-sided persons tend to be more attentive to detail and working methodically.

The Jungian assessment deals mostly with the ying-yang personality types: extroversion versus introversion, sensing a situation-based empirical affirmation versus using intuition based on the current environment, action based on thinking versus being based on feeling/emotions, and action based on judgment of options and alternatives versus basing action on perception based on prior knowledge and experience.

A-B indicators were a viewpoint of the 1940s and 1950s that held that people are Type A, Type B, or Type A/B. Type A person is one who is competitive, easily bored, impatient, in a rush, and possibly controversial. Type B is one who is relaxed, is easygoing, and maintains focus. The A–B type is able to present themselves as either. In today's highly competitive, fast-moving, and diverse world, a good leader should be able to present/mimic that trait that they are not normally to be fully understanding and be relative to the situation in a dynamic culture. The need for self-control is paramount to the level of self-possession.

The VARK Test is an assessment of how you learn: visual learners, aural learners, reading/writing learners, and kinesthetic learners. Visual learners learn by pictures, graphs, and spreadsheets. Aural learners learn by conversations and debate. Reading/Writing learners learn from written material, writing notes, summaries and e-mails/Internet, and Kinesthetic learners learn from practical exercises and hands-on approach. Knowing which type of learner you may be helps in becoming proficient in obtaining information that would be relevant to your leadership.

The New Enneagram Test has nine constructs of what is one's natural inclination toward behavior and how you will lead:

1) Reformer – Obedient; always tries to do the right thing; prefers others to get along with them. Tend to dictate terms to the group.
2) Helper – Seeks to engage in a supportive relationship to gain favor and acceptance. Tend to very interactive.
3) Thinker – The world is overstimulating and confusing; likes privacy to contemplate actions. Found to be most likely Type B. Tend to be direct, plain talkers with attention to detail and well thought out before they speak.
4) Skeptic – Very keen and curious Type A. Tend to being tactful and wary of irritating people.
5) Adventurer – Likes excitement and being the center of attention without taking responsibility. Tend be charismatic and hard to pin down.
6) Leader – Very assertive with a strong personality and direct. Tend to be self-reliant and unimpressed by other's opinions.
7) Peacemaker – Do not like to be in the spotlight or be in a prominent position. And prefer to "hide in plain sight." Tend to be a neutralizer with competing opinions [5].

In becoming a good leader for your practice and your staff, you must continually self-reflect and reevaluate your journey to become the best you.

Maxwell Maltz in his classic book *Psycho-Cybernetics* thoroughly discusses the need to self-reflect and reevaluate your leadership journey. He pointed out this reevaluation is much like a missile that must auto-correct many times to reach its destination [6]. Sometimes the missile goes off course to the left or the right only to make corrections to take it back on course. Likewise, as you go through leadership growth, through reflection and reevaluation, you will regain the proper course. But what is the proper course?

To find the right course to make you the best you, you can be, I can recommend following the 5 "Ds":

1) Dedication
2) Discipline
3) Decisiveness
4) Dependable
5) Demonstrable

To become the best version of your self, you must be dedicated to the pursuit of finding and developing that best version. This is not a pursuit of convenience but rather a dedicated way of life to constantly work toward a better you, even when the pursuit is difficult. Dedication is what pushes a leader through fear, criticism, doubt, delays, and obstacles with a can-do attitude, which leads you to success and inspires others along the way. As President Calvin Coolidge summed it up, "Nothing in this world can take the place of persistence. Talent will not: nothing is more common than unsuccessful men with talent. Genius will not; unrewarded genius is almost a proverb. Education will not: the world is full of educated derelicts. Persistence and determination alone are omnipotent."

Discipline of self may be the most important of the 5 "Ds". Through self-discipline you gain self-esteem and self-possession. Self-discipline also guides the many professional codes of ethics. Without self-discipline, small self-destructive acts or mannerisms will begin to invade that best version of your self you are trying to pursue and maintain. Such small acts over time begin to desensitize a developing leader and begin to be off course and down a slippery slope. As one becomes desensitized to a small unethical act or mannerism, increasingly larger such acts will have less awareness of their severity, thus limiting the best version of your self. Beware of immediate gratification that undermines your journey to living successfully. This is a very important reason for self-reflection that is needed to know thy self. The number of times and length of self-reflection needed will be dependent on the amount and severity of the self-destructive acts/mannerism encountered. Self-discipline also guides our choices in life. Following a dental practice guru (make more, get more, have more) in order to practice a certain way that may not be in a manner that would be best for you will interfere with your pursuit of the best you, you can be. Millions have been spent on how to make you a better practitioner (get new patients, how to close the deal, make more money), a better father or mother, or a better person. Everyone wants it fast and easy. Becoming the best version of your self takes time and a lot of effort. It is achieved by the choices you make. Making the right choices is based on your self-discipline, which leads to self-esteem and self-possession. This allows you to put control of your self, in your self, thereby allowing you to make the right choices to become the best version of your self. Without this self-discipline or self-control, you will become subservient to the many external negative influences. It will allow others to embed their mindset in you. The mental diet that you intentionally or unintentionally allow will affect the way you live. Constantly watching a reality show where arguing and fighting appear to be a normal way of life will desensitize you, if you do not have self-discipline. Hence, having self-discipline filters out the influences that which you would deem as self-destructive.

Decisiveness is very important since leadership is based on decisions. To be a wishy-washy and indecisive leader only gives uncertainty to the followers and eventually leads to chaos. Choices you make are yours forever and most times affect others. Many choices are based on past experiences and decision-making habits. If life is not progressing to living successfully, then reevaluate your attitude, your habits, and your choices. Most good decisions are made based on the information had at the time of the decision, the decision maker's experience, knowledge, and his or her most dominate thought immediately preceding the decision. Your actions are preceded and determined by your last most dominate thought. Whenever you make a decision, good or bad, take responsibility for it. You own it. If it is a good decision, a leader will give credit to those around him or her for making it work. If it is a bad decision, a leader will take full responsibility for it.

Dependability is very important because staff and patients will only follow your lead if they can depend on you to do the right thing. That includes keeping your word on various agreements, verbal or written. Many times people agree to do something but never had any intention for following through on that agreement. They were only trying to be "nice" or to take advantage of the other. A leader can easily lose their leadership position when it is found out that the leader never did what he or she said they would do, for example, misleading a staff member into thinking that they would receive a raise at a specified time but did not receive it, or a patient who was told that a discount would be given but was not. There are many small and large acts that can undermine a leader's standing.

Demonstrable leadership is a necessity of a true leader. As the saying goes, "If you talk the talk then you must walk the walk." A true leader would not ask one of his or her team members to do something they were not willing to do themselves. As a leader wanting the team to act a certain way with patients but you do not, the staff would have a hard time fulfilling your orders because you did not lead by example. Leading by example is possibly one of the best motivators in a small practice.

Many newly minted dentists have asked me how to become successful. My usual first answer is: how do you picture your self 5, 10, or even 20 years from now? Every great leader has personal goals set well into the future, and even if a goal is not met, they adjust and move forward in a positive manner to achieve their goals using their experiences as an education to move closer to being the best they can be. Although their goals might have changed, they are still set well into the future. Once a goal is met, a successful leader will immediately place new goals further into the future to maintain his or her successful course in life. A successful leader does not obtain a goal only to stop there and relish in the thought of succeeding; but rather, he or she immediately replaces that goal with another equally important. Great leaders understand that success of a goal is not an end point or destination but rather part of life's journey.

To illustrate this, look at a new dentist. Just out of school or residency, he or she will embark on the start of their professional career. Some may only see as far as hopefully getting a job, but others will see a future of building a practice. Once the practice is built up and going, he or she may become disenchanted with the mundane day-to-day practice of dentistry because he or she did not see any further goals other than to have a practice. Once having the practice they desired, they then turn to the goal of paying off the practice, which in turn once reached leaves the dentist unfulfilled. Production has reached a plateau, the procedures are become mundane, and the patients and staff are no longer invigorating. The next step is to work harder to plan for retirement, which in and of itself turns the enjoyment of practicing into a rut because of the repetitious workload of an experienced dentist and goals that have never really changed. They reach out to practice gurus or other third parties (many of which have never owned a dental practice) to find new ways to fulfill their want to be happy in their practice. What has happened is that change has occurred to them and the practice. They thought by setting end goals, and once the goal was achieved, it would bring them happiness. But it did not because life goals are not an end point but a stepping stone to finding the best version of your self. For a dentist to be successful at living, he or she must understand the importance of changing or expanding their goals as they are achieved throughout life. Without this understanding that life has changed, but their goals have not, they will be stuck in a rut of trying to become satisfied without success, because the goals have remained unchanged. Your practice like your life is a journey that must constantly evolve and grow. They will consider and describe themselves as successful, but are they? Many have regarded and even equated success with money. Money is only one facet or building block of success. Your practice is only one part of your life. There are other parts.

Being successful in business (your practice) is not the same as living successfully. Living successfully is much more rewarding and fulfilling and more successful by "having it all" as some would put it. It would be better described as being successful at living. To be successful at living, one must have a balance in your life that allows you to be "all that you can be." To achieve this balance, one must constantly work on what I call the 7 "F"s:

1) Family
2) Friends
3) Finances
4) Fitness
5) Formation
6) Fun
7) Faith

Family is very important, if not the most important, to the successful leader since it is the very best support system a leader can have. Family can also be detrimental to the leader if the family does not have the understanding that to be successful, there are some sacrifices that must be made. For example, a dentist's family is always upset at him or her because they are always late coming home due to patient emergencies. On the other hand, the dentist must not ignore the family's need for attention only to make more money. Conrad Hilton, founder of Hilton Hotels, had a very hard time with family commitments for the sake of building his empire. It was not until later in life that he realized the importance of family. I have never seen an armored truck filled with money in a funeral procession. I have always seen family and friends. Hence, there must be a balance in one's life with the family to achieve success.

Friends are always needed for feedback, guidance, and support. Almost everyone wants to have social interaction with others who appreciate who you are. Friends can have a positive or negative impact on you, depending on the choice of friends you have made. Friends can build you up, but they can also tear you down. Hence, choose friends wisely because of their huge impact on your life.

Finances are very important because it affords the other balancing pillars to be stable. Just making more and more money does not make the other pillars stronger. They must all be balanced. Having consulted many dentists with financial problems, I observed their lifestyle. Some dentists just out school or residency, having large education loans and even extended practice loans, live a lifestyle that is beyond their means simply because they think it is expected of them since they are dentists or because they believe they are entitled to it since they are dentists.

True Case (40)

There is also the possible problem of the competing spouses. Every time the dentist would invest in the practice with new equipment or adding a new employee, his wife would order new drapes and furniture or go out and buy herself jewelry to "make it even." This situation did not last long since two of the pillars were sacrificed: family and finances. The marriage eventually ended in divorce.

Fitness is very important for the obvious reason that you cannot do dentistry from a hospital bed. Dentistry is very physical and requires the dentist to maintain excellent physical condition. There are many experienced dentists that have had neck, back, and shoulder deterioration due to the repetitive movement required in dentistry. A dentist must use all their senses, both hands, neck, back, and even their feet to produce an income. It is imperative if you want to practice dentistry a long time because you enjoy it, you must exercise. I have been practicing over 40 years and will continue as long as I can since I truly enjoy my profession. Exercising (includes stretching, yoga, etc.) every day is a must. Dentistry being somewhat repetitive, you must try to adhere to proper ergonomic positioning of the patient, doctor, and assistant.

Formation is the education and training you have received and continue to build upon. It is not only the formal education and training but also the informal information gathered from mentors and others you admire or try to emulate that become part of you and add to who you are. Reading books, attending seminars, and listening to others express themselves all have an input on your improvement or your demise. Choosing those that have a positive impact should be paramount in what you watch or listen to.

Fun is very important because you must have relief from the stresses of work and life. Whether it is two weeks' vacations traveling the world, simply resting at home poolside, eating out, boating, fishing, hunting, or working in the yard, you need fun to unite with the family, to count your blessings, and to reignite your self. As the saying goes, "All work and no play makes Jack a dull boy."

Faith is very important because you must believe in something. Even the non-belief is a belief or mindset of what you believe in. All great leaders held a belief in something greater than mere humans. They believe that there are reasons other than self-serving to do good. A strong faith enables one to believe in a moral standard that is not egocentric and allows a leader to more easily reflect and improve one's self.

Keeping the 7 "F" pillars equally balanced and interconnected is not an easy task. At times one pillar may seem to falter, while another seems to be taking over. It is a constant job monitoring and making corrections like the missile mentioned before to maintain successful living. Hence you must always work toward improvement with constant self-awareness. Each of these areas of your life must have goals that are appropriate and attainable. Each of these areas should have 5-, 10-, and 20-year goals that will change and be adjusted because you will change in your life's journey. Achieving a true balance of these seven pillars will allow you to fulfill your success at living and being the best you, you can be.

When these seven pillars are not properly maintained, living successfully begins to unravel. It is usually due to choices one makes along the journey of life. Making choices affect the attitude one has. The more bad choices, the bigger chance of having a bad attitude, thereby not allowing you to attain the goal you sought. Therefore, if your goals are not being met, you do not like the goals you have chosen or it just didn't turn out the way you thought, then change your choices. Taking control of your choices controls attitude, self-esteem, self-possession, and how you see your self. Start working in a manner that will rebalance the seven pillars.

This is not easy without having appropriated time to spend on your self-awareness. As mentioned before, this is done by taking the time for some quiet time to allow the mind to synthesize all the input of your life. This quiet time is exactly that "Quiet" – meaning that there is no music, TV, or other background input. Some call this meditation. I prefer to call it a mindful time-out. It is the time you take to think and sort through your current life's situation. A constant reevaluation of where you are and where you are headed on all the "F" word levels must be done on a routine basis.

A simple way to do this is to reflect on Maxwell Maltz's meaning of success:

Sense of direction by setting proper goals for levels of your life.
Understanding situations and people who are in your life (family, staff, etc.).
Courage to do the right thing when it is hard to do.
Charity toward others in need (can be anonymously and equal to your abilities).
Esteem in both professional and personal life with positivity.
Self-confidence by being informed and knowledgeable through listening.
Self-acceptance by understanding oneself by taking quiet time-outs [7].

Therefore, you have a choice whether you want to just be successful or to be successful at living. It is not easy and takes a lot of time, patience, and practice.

To be a dental practice owner leader and taking your practice to the best it can be and not just an owner satisfied with mediocrity, you must adhere to 10 basic simple "How tos" as mentioned in Soupios and Mourdoukoutas's book *The Ten Golden Rules of Leadership* [8]:

1) Know thy self – A true understanding of yourself through an inventory of your self. Discover who you are and then build upon it. Who are you? What is it that you want to be or become (not just for business but for your life)? What do you want your life to stand for 5, 10, 20 years from now? You must have a good self-image, a positive self-image to have a good positive attitude towards others (including patients and staff) whereby you are positioning your self for living successfully.

True Case (41)

A young man once mentioned to me at a retreat that he would like to live his life in such a way that every person he had met throughout his life would like to come to his funeral because of the positive impact or positive influence he had on that person. Although this is a little morbid coming from a young man, it was his definition of how he wanted to live his life – positively influencing or impacting all the people that he would come in contact with throughout his life.

Knowing thy self is not the same for all. Some may feel the need to own several practices in a couple of states or feel the need to be a sole practitioner in a small village. Both may become successful at living. However, if the pursuit of a type of practice is based on external influences and not on the dentist's self, being successful at living will not be obtained.

2) Achieving power separates real leaders from pseudo-leaders in the use of that power. Being the owner of a dental practice, you automatically have power over your employees/staff. Will you use that power to be domineering over or supportive of the individual staff members? Will you be there to help each staff member to achieve their potential even if it means that you must fire them to head them in a new direction? Not every one you hire was destined to be in the dental field.

3) "We, not I" should be a center point in any discussion with or about the staff. Team building should always be the aim of capitalizing on the success of the practice. The dentist should not monopolize the practice's success by leaving the staff out of success acknowledgments. Constantly putting yourself first as the reason for the practice success and making it all about "ME," is a sure way to squash any team building efforts. You must share with the staff any and all praise patients place on you or the practice. This includes having the staff well paid within a good business structure and giving bonuses when indicated to give positive incentive and reward.

4) Understanding limitations as to what you can control and not control. Do not waste time and effort fighting uncontrollable situations. It is like fighting windmills because you are missing the opportunity to learn and move on. Taking full responsibility for controllable failures that may occur heightens your leadership credibility and integrity of your self. You are the leader and controllable failures would not happen if you had done your job right by properly training or educating the staff. Controllable failures are opportunities to learn and grow. It is what is called experience. As was mentioned before, all great leaders did experience failures from which he or she did learn from and made them better. Great leaders have managed to turn failures into a positive learning experience moving forward to achieve their goals.

5) Always be truthful and allow critics (this includes family, friends and staff) to test it. Being truthful is perhaps one of the most important traits on how to be a leader and become the best you, you can be. The veracity of your attitude, posturing, actions and statements is all important to your integrity as a true leader. That integrity is very important to withstand the test of critics who are always readily available in the midst of a leader. It is very hard to allow criticism; but, it is the best way to strengthen a leader's truthfulness and self-possession, which is control over your self. So, when a staff member questions a decision, be truthful, honest and sincere in your answer. You need to

understand that the staff member who is questioning or is critical may not know all the facts of the situation that led to the decision. Sometimes the criticism is right on target from which a good leader will take as an opportunity to improve and redirect back on course of becoming a better you.

6) Competition is the name of the game. To be competitive you must avoid mediocrity and be rid of any antagonistic destructive strifes in your practice and in your personal life. A great leader enjoys healthy competition from which the leader learns and yearns to do better. Competition raises the bar of achievement and makes your practice, your staff and your self better. As the bar is raised not all staff members may be able to move forward with the rest of the practice. Such situations bring out destructive antagonists, staff members that may try to undermine the progress since they cannot adjust to it. The dentist leader must keep the improvement of the practice and all the staff moving forward even if it means releasing an employee to seek a new employment opportunity elsewhere. This helps one to maintain balance toward successful living.

True Case (42)

A general dentist who owned a large multi-specialty fee-for-service practice had an orthodontist who did not want to incorporate newer orthodontic technologies (porcelain brackets/Invisalign) as they arrived, regardless of the large effort by all in the practice to encourage the orthodontist to do so. Because this was seen as a hindrance to the practice's ability to compete, the general dentist owner had to fire the orthodontist. He or she had become a destructive antagonist.

---

7) "Live by a higher code" (Aristotle). There is nothing more precious to a great leader than their integrity. The leader's reputation as one who lives by a higher code will always give others the basis on which they decide to follow. There have been many leaders throughout history that lacked a moral code and as a result are not regarded as leaders but rather dictators or despot. It is this trustworthiness and moral compass of their leader that makes a good leader great and become successful at living!

8) Critically evaluate information for origin, content and delivery. As the leader of your staff, patients and your self, any and all information that you encounter must be vetted as to the origin, content and delivery of that information. How trustworthy is it on all these levels? Before making any decision, you must make sure that you have all the information needed to make such a decision on any level personally or professionally. Not everything everyone tells you is the EXACT truth. It is human nature to re-phrase any communication one receives and

frame it as one believes to be the truth, when in agreement with such communication. Be sure not to blindly trust, but to verify all relied upon statements. Your integrity as the leader of the practice, staff and self depend on it.

9) Be careful of rationalizing your actions. It is a very slippery slope for a leader to start rationalizing poor decisions to maintain a self-created "I can do no wrong" attitude toward your practice, your patients and your self. Many good leaders have succumbed to the notion via their ego that they can do no wrong. Such a viewpoint is possibly one of the fastest ways to lose a great staff, ruin a great practice, and misguide your self.

True Case (43)

A dentist sold a very successful practice (large multi-specialty fee-for-service practice) to another dentist. The buying dentist appeared to be a very credible person with leadership qualities that the selling dentist thought would allow for the practice to continue for patients and staff. Shortly after the sale, specialists and staff members left due to an overbearing micromanaging new owner who thought he could do no wrong and still maintain the practice as it was. The buying dentist was told many times by the many specialists and some of the long-term (20 years') staff that the "his way or the highway" attitude will not work in such a large practice and should be working together for the betterment of all (specialists and staff). Within in six months all was lost.

---

10) Your leadership determines your fate. You have choices and as a leader, you will make many choices for your practice, your staff, and your self that once made are yours forever. It is the great leader that when making a choice, whether it results in a good or a bad outcome, will learn from it and make more good choices and refrain from bad choices. That is why great leaders are made and not just a result of fate.

There is one more concern that few care to discuss in obtaining true leadership of self: burnout.

Maintaining a high level of leadership, communication, and engagement at all levels may become difficult to keep lively over a long period of time. The core of the burnout experience is emotional exhaustion secondary to workloads and work demands, constrained resources, and lack of interpersonal support at any level within the 7 "Fs."

In 2017, 37% of adults in the United States stated their stress level had increased over the past year, a rise from previous years. It was found that 18% of those with management responsibilities often felt stressed. It was also found, as of 2016, that 31.4% of physicians had feelings of burnout [9]. Burnout is real and affects many at different stages of their professional career and in different ways. Burnout is not a simple result of long hours. The cynicism, depression, and lethargy of burnout can occur when you are not in control of how you carry out your job, when you are working toward goals that do not resonate with you, and when you lack social (and family) support [10]. In a study of burnout among new dentists, practice management (PM) issues that correlated to high levels of stress included law and insurance matters, practice organization, and staff management [11]. Another study focusing on work stressors of dentists reported in 1998 that time management and coping with difficult patients were major factors [11]. Hence, there becomes an imbalance of the 7 "Fs".

So how do you know when you are headed to the edge of burnout? Here are possibly nine items that you can review during your self-reflection time. No texting. No Internet. Just you and your introspective practice of self-reflection.

1) Your motivation has faded. Your passion to lead has vaporized or has become self-centered.
2) Your main emotion is "numbness" – you no longer feel the highs or the lows. If you just don't care anymore, you are then on the edge of numbness.
3) People drain you. Many people do that in the best of times. But when you no longer find anyone to energize you or to talk to, you feel drained.
4) Little things make you disproportionately angry. You start losing your cool over the littlest of things.
5) You're becoming cynical. Having a negative, doubting mindset is a clear sign that you are on the edge of burnout.
6) Your productivity is dropping. You might be working more hours but the outcome value is less. Everything takes longer and results in less.
7) You're self-medicating. This could be overeating, drinking, impulsive spending, or even working more. These all add to the spiral into burnout.
8) You don't laugh anymore. Nothing seems funny or at its worst, you begin to resent people who enjoy life.
9) Sleep and time off no longer refuel you. Sometimes a good night sleep or a couple of weeks on vacation may do the job. But when you take time off and find that you come back with the same angst and feelings, you need to address your burnout issues [12].

If you find your self in several of the above situations, take the giant step and address it. Physicians who actively nurture and protect their personal and professional well-being on all levels – physical, emotional, psychological, and spiritual (again fulfilling the 7 "Fs") – are more likely to prevent or at least to mitigate it's consequences [10]. Take a quiet moment to seek the "Why?" you are headed toward or already burned out. If you are able to limit down the reason for your spiral into burnout, take appropriate action to confront it. Recovering from burnout is a slow process that must be worked on daily. Below are six strategies that when taken alone or as a composite may help relieve or even redirect you away from burnout:

1) You can even keep a stress diary to help direct you to the "Why?." Once identified, seek a way to relieve that stress. This might involve delegating the items giving you stress. It may mean seeking a mentor for direction or re-prioritizing your life to begin to live life successfully and get back to balancing the 7 "Fs".

2) Redirect your focus on your self. Start an exercise program not just for the body but also for the mind. Not only does regular exercise help to reduce stress, but it also boosts your mood, improves your overall health, and enhances your quality of life. Be sure you are getting enough sleep, eat well, and be sure to drink water. Work overloads tend to overtake the needed attention to your well-being. If you are constantly waking up during the night to try and remember something for the next day or have that "light bulb" thought from the subconscious, I advise you to get a piece of paper and a pen, and write down the thought that is keeping you awake or has just sprung forth. Putting it on paper relieves you of constantly waking up and trying to remember it. Eating good food is paramount in maintaining a healthy body and mind. Get rid of the snack food, microwaved dinners, and energy drinks. Be sure to hydrate well throughout the day. Mentally, get involved in activities outside of the areas causing the symptoms of burnout and turn your attention away from that stress source. Getting involved in family, community service, sports, church, synagogue, or temple. These might sound obvious, but busy professionals often ignore their most basic needs. Instead, they take care of others and their responsibilities far more than they take care of themselves.

3) Take a vacation or leave of absence. Not just a long weekend but a real vacation. Although not always financially possible, even a staycation for a week away from the daily work routine might be found to be helpful. Either going on a vacation away or a staycation at home, *all* contact with work should be severed. No phone calls, e-mails, or texting! You are away! When I was just starting out, married and have two little children, with very little discretionary money, we would take a staycation for one week. We would go out in the morning and go to local (within a day's drive) attractions and not come home till the early evening.

4) Reassess your goals. You must not only constantly mentally check on your progress toward your goals but also check to see if those previously set goals are still presently applicable. Are your values still intact or have they changed for the better or the worse? Every successful leader has had to reset their goals and reevaluate their current set of values to meet their current situation and improve it.

5) Say "No," politely. Leaders are invariably asked to help solve problems, to help with others responsibilities and commitments, and to lend leadership

to a group, cause, or endeavor. Not everyone has the want or the attributes to constantly give and/or take on more responsibilities. Overload in helping others will take its toll on your ability to live life successfully – not to become a recluse, but to acknowledge the intrusion of always saying "Yes" on the family, practice, and your self.

6) Practice positive thinking. Try thinking of something positive before you get out of bed each morning. Or, at the end of the day, think back to one great thing that you did at work or at home. You deserve to celebrate even small accomplishments. These celebrations can help you rediscover joy and meaning in your work again. It is very important to become honed in the use of affirmations. Affirmations are positive statements about the future. They also help you visualize and believe in what you are doing. Get in the habit of a daily affirmation followed by a visualization of that thought. If you can visualize it, and keep that visualization alive, it will become a dominate thought. Our actions and choices are based on our last most dominate thought. This exercise will allow the visualization of your affirmation to become a materialization and manifestation of that thought process. Therefore, your morning positive affirmation will lead you to positive choices that in turn lead to be successful at living. This is an exercise that must be regularly done in small steps to move from a negative burned-out mindset to a vibrant positive can-do attitude [13].

Keeping a positive outlook no matter the situation can be best described by Admiral Nimitz's comments when he was given a boat tour of the destruction wrought on Pearl Harbor by the Japanese. Big sunken battleships and Navy vessels cluttered the waters everywhere you looked.

True Case (44)

As the tour boat returned to dock, the young helmsman of the boat asked, "Well Admiral, what do you think after seeing all this destruction?" Admiral Nimitz's reply shocked everyone within the sound of his voice. Admiral Nimitz said, "The Japanese made three of the biggest mistakes an attack force could ever make, or God was taking care of America. Which do you think it was?"

Shocked and surprised, the young helmsman asked, "What do mean by saying the Japanese made the three biggest mistakes an attack force ever made?" Nimitz explained:

Mistake number 1: The Japanese attacked on Sunday morning. Nine out of every 10 crewmen of those ships were ashore on leave. If those same ships had been lured to sea and been sunk, we would have lost 38 000 men instead of 3800.

Mistake number 2: When the Japanese saw all those battleships lined in a row, they got so carried away sinking those battleships, and they never once bombed our dry docks opposite those ships. If they had destroyed our dry docks, we would have had to tow every one of those ships to America to be repaired. As it is now, the ships are in shallow water and can be raised. One tug can pull them over to the dry docks, and we can have them repaired and at sea by the time we could have towed them to America. And I already have crews ashore anxious to man those ships.

Mistake number 3: Every drop of fuel in the Pacific theater of war is on top of the ground storage tanks five miles away over that hill. One attack plane could have strafed those tanks and destroyed our fuel supply. That's why I say the Japanese made three of the biggest mistakes an attack force could make or God was taking care of America.

Any way you look at it, Admiral Nimitz was able to see a silver lining in a situation and circumstance where everyone else saw only despair and defeatism [14]. That is a "can-do" positive leadership.

To sum up success, H. Jackson Brown Jr. gives 21 suggestions for success. Note there is only one mention of money.

Marry the right person. This one decision will determine 90% of your happiness or misery.
Work at something you enjoy and that's worthy of your time and talent.
Give people more than they expect and do it cheerfully.
Become the most positive and enthusiastic person you know.
Be forgiving of yourself and others.
Be generous.
Have a grateful heart.
Persistence, persistence, persistence.
Discipline yourself to save money on even the modest salary.
Treat everyone you meet like you want to be treated.
Commit yourself to constant improvement.
Commit yourself to quality.
Understand that happiness is not based on possessions, power, or prestige, but on relationships with people you love and respect.
Be loyal.
Be honest.
Be a self-starter.
Be decisive even if it means you'll sometimes be wrong.
Stop blaming others. Take responsibility for every area of your life.
Be bold and courageous. When you look back on your life, you'll regret things you didn't do more than the ones you did.
Take good care of those you love.
Don't do anything that wouldn't make your Mom proud.

"Don't just light up your life, IGNITE it!!"
Joseph P. Graskemper

References

1 Belitz, J. (2006). *Success: Full Thinking*, 19. Pen & Publish.
2 Ledlow, G.R. and Coppola, M.N. (2011). *Leadership for Health Professionals*, 25. Sudbury, MA: Jones and Bartlett Learning.
3 Ledlow, G.R. and Coppola, M.N. (2011). *Leadership for Health Professionals*, 28. Sudbury, MA: Jones and Bartlett Learning.
4 Ledlow, G.R. and Coppola, M.N. (2011). *Leadership for Health Professionals*, 29. Sudbury, MA: Jones and Bartlett Learning.
5 Ledlow, G.R. and Coppola, M.N. (2011). *Leadership for Health Professionals*, 29–32. Sudbury, MA: Jones and Bartlett Learning.
6 Maltz, M. (1960). *Psycho-cybernetics*, 18. New York: Pocket Books.
7 Maltz, M. (1960). *Psycho-cybernetics*, 113. New York: Pocket Books.
8 Soupios, M.A. and Mourdoukoutas, P. (2015). *The Ten Golden Rules of Leadership*, 126–127. New York: American Management Association.
9 https://www.statista.com/topics/2099/stress-and-burnout/ (accessed 19 June 2018).
10 Balch, C., Freischlag, J., and Shanafelt, T. (2009). Stress and burnout among surgeons. *Achieves of Surgery Journal* 144 (4): 373.
11 Schonwetter, D. and Schwartz, B. (2018). Comparing practice management courses in Canadian dental schools. *Journal of Dental Education* 82 (5): 502.
12 Nieuwhof, C. (2013). 9 Signs You're Burning Out in Leadership. https://careynieuwhof.com/9-signs-youre-burning-out-in-leadership/ (accessed 19 June 2018).
13 (a) Cherniss, D. (1991). Long-term consequences of burnout: an exploratory study. *Journal of Organizational Behaviour* 13 (1). (b)Leiter, M.P. (1992). Coping patterns as predictors of burnout: the function of control and escapist coping patterns. *Journal of Organizational Behaviour* 12 (2); (c) Penedo, F.J. and Dahn, J.R. (2005). Exercise and well-being: a review of mental and physical health benefits associated with physical activity. *Current Opinion in Psychiatry* 18 (2); (d) https://www.mindtools.com/pages/article/recovering-from-burnout.htm (accessed 19 June 2018).
14 Admiral Chester Nimitz (1942). Reflections on Pearl Harbor. https://seekingalpha.com/instablog/388783-christopher-menkin/242946-reflections-on-pearl-harbor-by-admiral-chester-nimitz (accessed 23 June 2018).

Index

Leadership and Communication in Dentistry, First Edition. Joseph P. Graskemper.
© 2019 John Wiley & Sons, Inc. Published 2019 by John Wiley & Sons, Inc.